A SURGEON'S (

SHOULDER

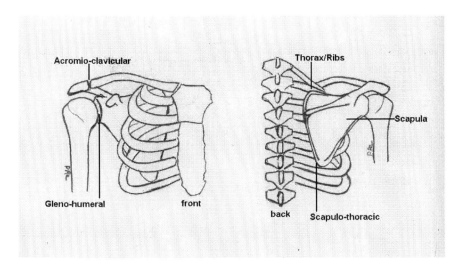

Acromio-clavicular

Gleno-humeral

front

Thorax/Ribs

Scapula

back   Scapulo-thoracic

by Paul Re M.D.

illustrated by Paul Re M.D.

To my Family

Their love for and dedication to me

Allows me to be dedicated to my profession

"State of the art book on shoulder problems and their treatment. This book is an excellent education source for patients, students, residents, therapist and doctors. Dr. Re writes in a conversational way that makes complex injuries simple to understand. A great addition to the conversation on the shoulder."

Gregory T. Altman M.D.

Clinical Associate Professor Orthopedic Surgery

Temple University School of Medicine

Vice Chairman Department of Orthopedic Surgery

Allegheny General Hospital

Team Physician Pittsburgh Pirates

DISCLAIMER

The contents of this book are for informational purposes only. It is not medical advice or diagnosis. It is not intended to be a substitute for professional medical exam, advice, diagnosis or treatment. Always seek the advice of a qualified medical health care provider for any condition you have. Never disregard any medical advice or delay in seeking it because of something you have read in this book.

The reading of this book does not create any patient physician relationship. It is not a substitute for professional diagnosis and treatment. We are not responsible and have no liability for any damages, loss, injury or lability whatsoever suffered as a result of your reliance on the information contained in the book.

The exercises, images and programs discussed in this book are not a substitute for medical advice. Always consult a medical professional before starting a new medicine, work out or physical therapy program. We are not responsible for any injury suffered by performing these exercises or programs.

This book contains information, images and exercises that are only intended to make the reader better informed consumers of health care. Always consult your health care provider for evaluation and treatment of your specific issue.

The best way to cure a shoulder problem is to avoid it. Keep your shoulder flexible and in a posture that limits the risk for injury. Focus on obtaining and maintaining good and proper shoulder mechanics.

Keep your shoulder and shoulder blades back and down.

INTRODUCTION

The shoulder is one of the most versatile joints in the body, and it has a range of motion greater than any other joint. However, the same motion that its joints give it, places the shoulder at risk for injury.

A joint is where two bones of the body meet; a junction that allows for movement. A joint is also called an articulation. Major joints are usually found at the end portions of long bones in our body. For the hip it is at the end our thigh bone (femur), and for our knee, it is at the top of the shin bone, (tibia). The shoulder is where our upper arm bone, the humerus, articulates with the wing bone (the scapula). Where these bones meet, the surface of the bone is covered with a smooth, gliding surface called articular cartilage. This articular cartilage allows for near frictionless motion.

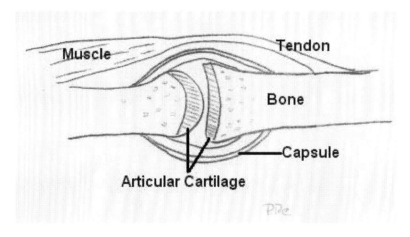

FIGURE 1

Each joint has its own distinct shape, and this shape defines its motion as well as its stability. Other factors that define a joint's movement and stability are the structures that surround that joint including the capsule, ligaments, and muscles. The capsule is a sheet like tissue that connects the two bones at a joint and offers some stability. A ligament is a more robust, thicken cord like tissue that also connects the two bones at a joint and gives a stronger connection. The capsule and ligaments do not actively move and are known as static stabilizers of the joint. The muscles through their contraction and strength give what is known as a dynamic stabilization to the joint. (figure 1)

The joint's movement and stability are related to the shape of the surfaces where they meet, the pliability and flexibility of the capsule that surrounds it, the number and strength of the ligaments connecting the two articulating bones, and the strength of the muscles that act across that joint. So you can see that there are many factors that affect one joint's stability relative to another joint.

The more stable a joint is, the less motion it has. Conversely, the more motion a joint is capable of achieving, the more inherently unstable it is. In addition, the more motion a joint has, the more it depends upon its capsule, its ligaments and its muscles to give it stability.

The shoulder, where the top of the humerus bone articulates with the glenoid surface of the scapula, has among the largest range of motions of all joints in the body. As a result, it is also one of the most unstable and most frequently dislocated joints in the body. Let's compare it to two other major joints in the body: the hip and the knee.

THE HIP

The hip is a ball and socket joint. (figure 2) It is a stable form for a joint to have. The stability of the ball and socket joint is a function of a couple of things but mostly how much the socket covers the ball. Doctors often make reference to, 'how deep the socket is.' Basically, the deeper the socket is, the more it covers the ball and thus the more stable the joint it. As a result of this increased coverage, the joint has less motion.

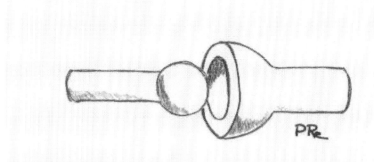

FIGURE 2

The ball and socket shape gives it excellent inherent stability, good load characteristics in multiple planes, but its range of motion in a three-dimensional plane is limited.

As the old song goes, the foot bone is connected to the shin bone, the shin bone is connected to the knee bone, the knee bone is connected to the hip bone, and the hip bone is connected to the pelvis bone... Well the hip is the major joint that connects the leg to the body. In particular, with the foot being at the end of the leg, the hip's main purpose is to connect the foot to the body, allow us to move the foot away from our body and walk or run. Moving that foot away from our body and then loading that foot and leg with our weight, requires a very strong and stable joint and that is why our hip is inherently stable. We need it to be in order to support our weight when we move. We don't need much motion for that function.

In one plane the hip has flexion and extension: it brings the leg in front of the body and up to the belly as well as backwards behind the axial line of the spine. The ability to flex up to our belly gives us the ability to climb.

In another plane it has abduction and adduction: it brings the leg out to the side and laterally away from the axial skeleton, as well as in toward the center and towards the axial skeleton. This gives us side to side stability and balance.

In the last plane the hip has external and internal rotation, which is rotating the leg, outwards and inwards about the axial axis of the hip. This gives us stability on uneven surfaces.

While the hip has a good range of motion, it is still quite limited. The shape of the hip socket limits the hip to a 'cone' of motion much smaller than a half of a hemisphere. Again in this case, range of motion is being sacrificed for stability. (figure 3)

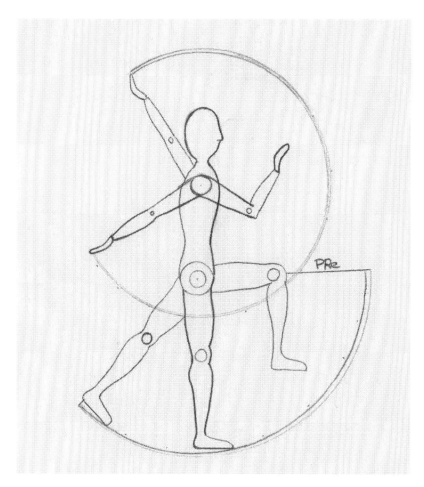

FIGURE 3

18

THE KNEE

The knee is another important joint of the lower extremity. One of its main purposes is to lift the foot off the ground, making walking, climbing, running all possible. It is what is called a hinge joint. (figure 4)

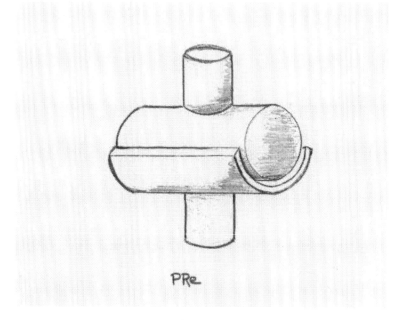

PRe

FIGURE 4

While it does have very minor rotational motion and even much less side-to-side motion, for all intents and purposes it really functions in one plane, which is flexion and extension. Once again, with its main purpose forward and backward motion, elevating the foot off the ground to make climbing and walking possible. It has

19

sacrificed motion in other planes to maximize motion in one plane and stability in that motion.

THE SHOULDER

Let's take a look at the shoulder. The shoulder is also a ball and socket joint, but the socket is incredibly shallow and the ball is very uncovered. So as you have already figured out, the shoulder has a great amount of motion but is very unstable.

In order to understand the shoulder, we need to first understand the purpose of the shoulder or what the shoulder allows us to do. The purpose of the shoulder is to place the hand in the space around our body. (figure 5) The hand, at the end of the arm, is connected to our body at the shoulder. In other words, the shoulder is the connection of the hand to the chest and body. The shoulder is the platform that allows the hand to be used effectively.

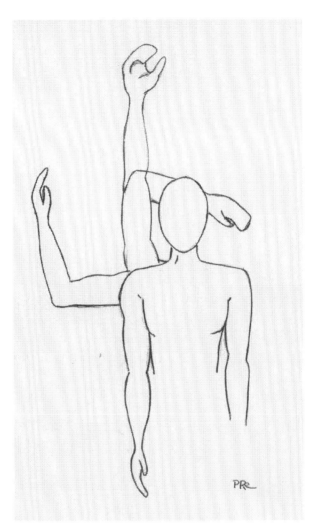

FIGURE 5

Being a biped, that is that we walk upright on our feet and legs, has freed our upper extremities for use other than walking on them. Once used mostly for locomotion, as in quadrupeds like horses, dogs and other four-legged mammals, our upper extremities are no longer front legs, they are arms. And since they are no longer legs, our shoulders don't have to be as stable as hips. So our shoulders have developed more motion to allow us to place our hands in a wider array of positions away from our body. It allows us to reach, grab, climb, and use tools.

Our body has sacrificed the speed and stability that comes from four legs in order to use our upper limbs for more intricate tasks. This potential evolved along with our brain's cognitive ability to use these specialized limbs. This development raises the question of whether the evolution of the brain's cognitive ability selected for specialized limbs or the selection of specialized limbs trained the brain and encouraged and promoted cognitive ability. Interestingly, they most likely evolved in concert with each other.

It is this transition from quadruped to biped ambulation that has made our hips more stable and shoulders less so. In examining the capsular fibrous strand orientation of the hip we see that as the hip has changed from a quadruped orientation to a biped orientation, the femoral head (ball) in relation to the acetabulum (socket) has become more extended as we evolved an upright stance, and thereby the capsular fibrous orientation has twisted. (figure 6)

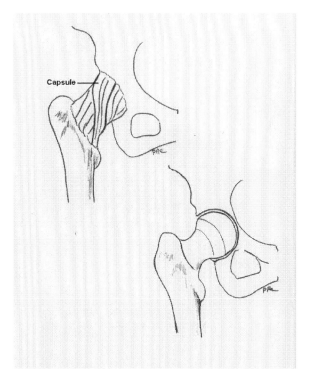

FIGURE 6

This twisting of the capsule makes the hip joint more stable. As one ambulates and flexes the hip, the capsule 'untwists,' but when standing still and upright, a position in which we require the most stability to make upright posture possible, the hip capsule returns to the twisted/ coiled, stable orientation.

On the other hand, the shoulder joint typically rests in the uncoiled/ untwisted position with the arm by the side, but when lifting the arm up, the capsule becomes more twisted and thereby more stable as we place our hand away from our body. (figure 7)

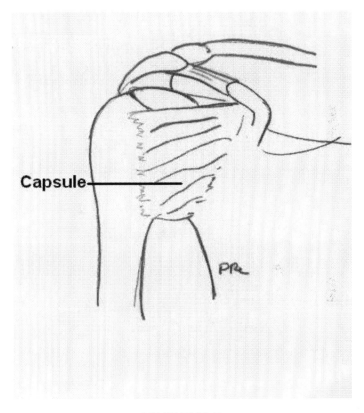

FIGURE 7

Our success as humans has been in large part due to the ability to use our upper extremities and in particular our hands, and even more precisely, our opposable thumb, for specialized tasks. The shoulder is the platform for the potential of the hand's position. Imagine your shoulder as a center point, extend your elbow, hand and fingers fully, now rotate your arm in all directions. You have now created a potential sphere of motion that your shoulder can place your hand in, in order to perform a task. It is almost a complete full sphere. Flexing your elbow allows the hand to be placed to any point within that sphere, but it is the shoulder that sets that platform. (figure 3,5)

In summary, the shoulder is a ball and socket joint. The socket is shallow; leaving the ball uncovered which gives it more motion but less stability. The capsule around the shoulder is untwisted when the arm is by our side but it twists when the arm is moved. This twisting gives it more stability when lifting the arm and hand away from the body. The muscles around the shoulder joint also play a significant role in stabilizing the shoulder. We will examine that later.

THE SHOULDER JOINT IN DETAIL

From a functional standpoint, the shoulder really isn't one joint, rather it is three joints working together. The way the shoulder achieves all of its motion is through the combination of these three major joints: the Gleno-humeral, the Acromio-clavicular, and the Scapulo-thoracic Joints. (figure 8). Let's examine each more closely.

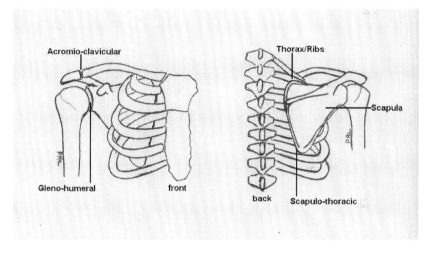

FIGURE 8

The Gleno-humeral Joint is the main area of motion. It is where the top of the upper arm, the humeral head articulates with the scapula. The part of the scapula that the humeral head articulates with is the glenoid.

The Acromio-clavicular Joint, sometimes simply

called the 'AC Joint,' is how the scapula, connects to the body. The clavicle is the thin 'S' shaped bone on the front of your upper chest. It connects to your body at the rib cage's sternum and then to your scapula at the part of the scapula called the acromion. Its purpose is to attach the shoulder to the body by a bony joint connection and it keeps your scapulas back and prevents them from collapsing forward. Keeping your scapulas back is a very important factor in shoulder function and injury prevention.

The scapula-thoracic joint is not a true articular joint, because where these two areas meet there is not any articular cartilage. It is where the scapula, sits on the back of your rib cage (the thorax). The scapula does move up and down and rotate on the thorax but there is no cartilage there, just muscle and bursa. This joint is important for the movement of the wing bone up and down, forward and back. The muscles that connect the scapula to the thorax and spine are incredibly important for the stabilization of the shoulder and allowing the hand to be used effectively.

THE GLENO-HUMERAL JOINT

It is the Gleno-humeral joint that most people consider the shoulder and it is also where most of the motion comes from. This is the ball in socket we have been discussing. As we talked about, the socket is shallow, it is more dish like in shape. An analogy often used is that the Gleno-humeral joint looks like a golf ball on a golf tee. (figure 9)

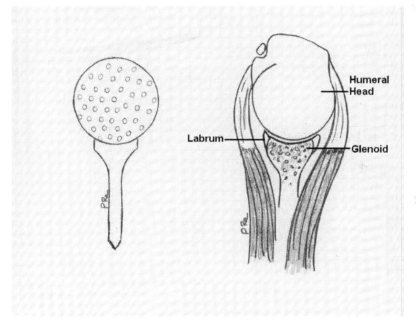

FIGURE 9

The Gleno-humeral joint is where the upper arm (the humerus) connects to the scapula.

The ball at the top of the humerus is the humeral

head. The rounded smooth top is covered with articular cartilage that provides a low friction gliding surface for smooth motion. Below this are bony protuberances, called the tuberosities, to which the rotator cuff muscles attach. Below this, other major muscles like the Deltoid and the Pectoralis Major and the Teres Major attach. (figure 10)

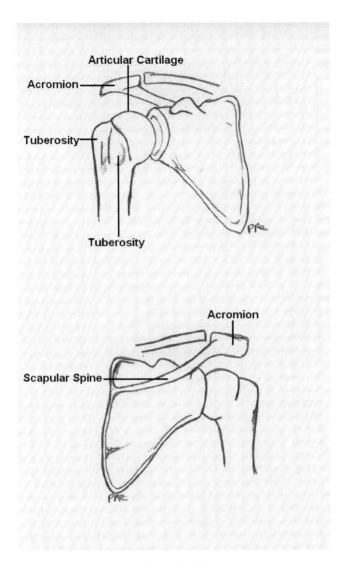

Articular Cartilage

Acromion

Tuberosity

Tuberosity

Acromion

Scapular Spine

FIGURE 10

The Scapula is what most people call the 'wing bone,' or 'shoulder blade.' It is upside down, triangular in shape and sits on your back chest wall. At the lateral point, farthest from the midline of the body, is the socket for the humerus to articulate with. The socket is called the glenoid. As a socket, the glenoid is shallow in depth. It anatomically looks like a golf ball (the head of the humerus) sitting on a golf tee (the glenoid). (figure 9)

Like the humeral head, the glenoid socket is also covered with articular gliding cartilage. Along the rim of the glenoid is another type of cartilage called the labrum. The labrum serves two main purposes, first it extends the surface of the glenoid joint to aid in stabilization by deepening the socket depth of the glenoid, and second it is the place to which the joint capsule attaches. (figure 11)

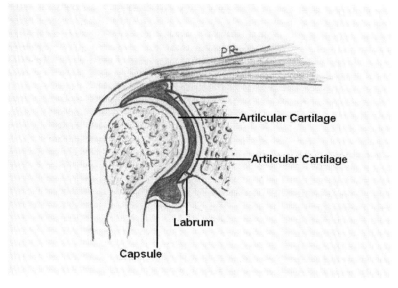

FIGURE 11

Extending back off the scapula is the scapular spine (figure 8,10). The scapular spine divides a couple of the rotator cuff muscles into compartments and also provides a spot for other scapular stabilizing muscles to attach. At the lateral part of the scapular spine is a bigger extending piece of bone. This thickened portion of the scapular spine then hooks superiorly and anteriorly forming the acromion, or roof, of the shoulder. (figure 10)

The outside edge of the acromion is where the Deltoid muscle attaches. The inside edge is where the clavicle articulates at the Acromio-clavicular joint (AC Joint). The underside of the acromion is where bone spurs often arise and is the source of pathology for a lot of people.

Starting at the center of the Gleno-humeral joint is the articular gliding cartilage. Extending outward, the next structure we come across is the joint capsule. (figure 12)

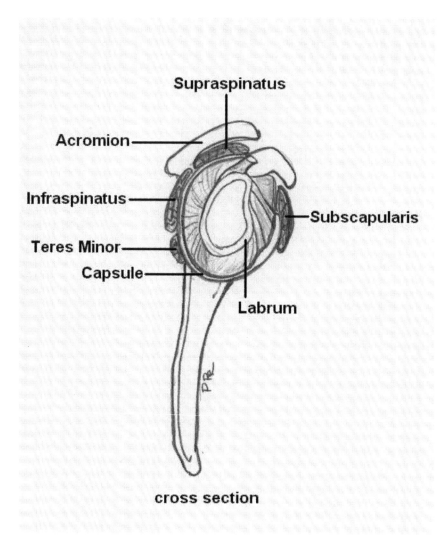

Supraspinatus

Acromion

Infraspinatus

Teres Minor

Capsule

Subscapularis

Labrum

cross section

FIGURE 12

The joint capsule starts at the edge of the articular cartilage of the humerus and connects to the labrum of the glenoid. (figures 11, 12) It is comprised of ligaments that attach one bone to another. This joint capsule is the primary stabilizer of the Gleno-humeral joint. It is called a 'static stabilizer' as it doesn't move on its own and acts like an anchor line or checkrein.

The Rotator Cuff is the group of muscles that help center and stabilize the Gleno-humeral joint. It is made up of a group of four muscles and tendons. The rotator cuff muscles start on the scapula, cross the Gleno-humeral joint and insert on the proximal humerus' tuberosities as tendons. They consist of the Subscapularis, the Supraspinatus, the Infraspinatus and the Teres Minor. (figure 13) They surround the humeral head.

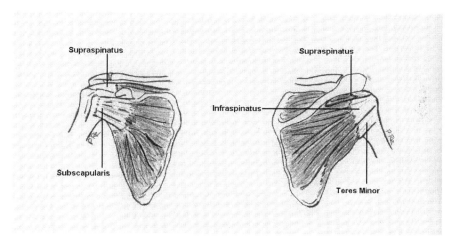

FIGURE 13

The rotator cuff tendons connect the rotator cuff muscle to the humeral head. The muscles each start distinctly and independently, and as they turn into tendons, they join together and insert onto the humerus. This joining together or confluence of the tendons is where the term 'cuff' comes from: a cuff of tendons surrounding the humeral head. Like a cuff at the end of your sleeve draping over your wrist, this cuff of tendons drapes over the humeral head. Each muscle can independently contract and move its tendon and the bone it's connected to. However, because all these tendons are connected and joined together at the 'cuff', a muscle can secondarily affect the tendon of another muscle. This is why some people don't know they have a small rotator cuff tear. Even though there may be a small tear in one of their rotator cuff tendons, the other muscles and tendons that are still attached can sometimes compensate for the torn portion in low demand situations.

This phenomenon is further helped by an anatomical thickening within the rotator cuff tendons called the 'rotator cuff cable.' This thickened cord strengthens the tendons' connection to each other and distributes stress across the rotator cuff cable. Roughly, it attaches to the humerus at the leading edge of the Subscapularis, arcs postero-medially and then back to the humerus again, attaching near the trailing edge of the Infraspinatus. A small tear of the tendon within the portion of the tendon bounded by the cable can go unrecognized in some low demand situations. The reason for this is that even though this portion of the supraspinatus tendon may be torn, the muscle is still attached to the cable next to it. In addition, the other rotator cuff muscles are also indirectly attached to this cable and together can move the shoulder through the cable. (figure 14)

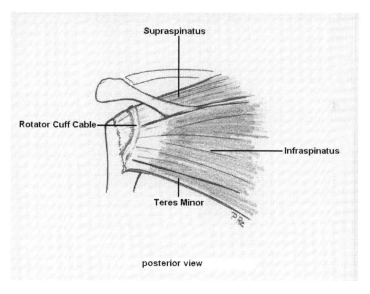

FIGURE 14

This cable joining the tendons is comparable to that of a suspension bridge cable and the distribution of the force of the road hanging from it. On the bridge, the load is distributed to the whole suspension cable by the tie cables that attach the road to the suspension cable. This force coupling helps to strengthen the construct by sharing the load and not overloading one portion.

Similarly, the 'cable' within the rotator cuff tendon shares the work load, translating the coupled forces of tendons, sometimes compensating for a small tear. This can occur if the intact muscles are strong, balanced and attached to the other. (figure 15)

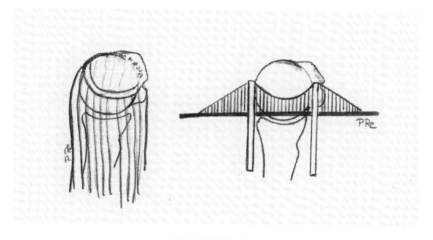

FIGURE 15

The purpose of the rotator cuff is three fold:

First, it rotates the humeral head within the glenoid socket, but the larger muscles that surround the shoulder such as the Deltoid, the Pectoralis and Teres Major perform the majority of heavy lifting.

Second, the rotator cuff balances the movement of these muscles and constantly centers the humeral head within the glenoid socket. That is, it keeps the center of rotation of the Gleno-humeral joint in a near constant place and within a few millimeters of normal. This allows the moment arm of the larger muscles to remain at their optimal length so they can work most efficiently.

Third, the balancing of these muscles act as a secondary stabilizer of the Gleno-humeral joint. Since the capsule is loose and allows for motion between the humeral head and glenoid, the rotator cuff fires and works to stabilize the shoulder and lock it in place. The rotator cuff is called a 'dynamic stabilizer' as it is constantly firing and moving to achieve stability, while the capsule is a 'static' stabilizer, as it has no inherent motion or contractile ability.

The Deltoid is one of the major muscles of the shoulder. It starts on the top of the scapula at a place called the acromion. The acromion is a bony roof that covers the top of the Gleno-humeral joint and the supraspinatus travels beneath it. The Deltoid starts at the edge of the acromion, travels downward around the rotator cuff tendons and inserts onto the upper humerus about 15 centimeters below the acromion. The Deltoid is the 'work horse' of the shoulder and is mainly responsible for the elevation of the humerus. (figure 20)

The acromion, sticking out over the joint, gives the Deltoid a better lever arm to work with. In every joint there exists a center of rotation point. That is the point about which all motion rotates. Any object that rotates has a center or axis of rotation. For example, a child spinning a baton in her hand has the center of rotation where her hand holds the baton.

A wrench is considered to have an axis of rotation at the center point of the nut that it is tightening or loosening. Anyone who has loosened a nut using a wrench knows that the longer the wrench is, the easier it is to use. That is because the farther the force used to move about that axis of rotation is away from that axis, the more efficient that force is. (figure 16) This principle is also seen in levers. 'Give me a lever long enough and a fulcrum on which to place it, and I shall move the world.'-Archimedes. In the body we see many boney protuberances onto which muscles attach. These protuberances lengthen the distance that the levers are away from the center of rotation to help the muscle work better.

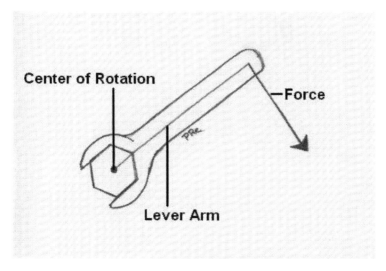

FIGURE 16

For the Gleno-humeral joint, the center of rotation is roughly in the center of the humeral head. This center of rotation of the humeral head lines up with the center of the glenoid socket. During range of motion of the shoulder, the rotator cuff keeps the center of rotation of the humeral head in the center of the glenoid (socket) and a safe distance away from the acromion.

The importance of this fact cannot be understated, for it is this constant distance away from the acromion that allows the Deltoid to function most efficiently and prevents damage to the tendons by avoiding contact with the acromion. The rotator cuff keeps the humeral head in position in the socket and thereby keeps the Deltoid at its optimal length.

The Deltoid muscle works as a lever on the shoulder and is effective because the acromion hangs over the Gleno-humeral joint and the edge of the acromion is set away from the center of rotation of the Gleno-humeral joint.

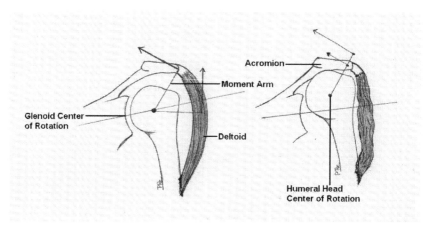

FIGURE 17

If the center of rotation of the Gleno-humeral joint rises superiorly a couple of things happen.

The first is that it shortens and weakens the moment arm of the Deltoid muscle, thereby making it more difficult to raise the arm. (figure 17)

The second is that it shortens the optimal length of the Deltoid muscle. Muscles function most efficiently when they are their appropriate length. There is only a limited and defined amount that these muscles can contract and shorten. Actinomycin is the protein complex responsible for contracting muscles. Actin is like a rachet that engages the Myosin which shortens/contracts the muscle.

If the muscle is slack, then the Actinomycin complexes cannot shorten enough to take up the slack, thereby making the muscle's contraction weaker, less effective and possibly useless.

As a comparison, imagine two people standing ten feet apart holding a ten-foot piece of rope taut. Now assume that they each can pull 1 foot length of rope, then if either of them pulls on the rope, the rope and the other person would move. This time imagine the same situation but the two people are now only nine feet apart. If one person pulls one foot of rope, the other person won't move because that person's pulling only took up the one-foot slack in the rope. If the other person pulls as well, then a resultant force will be translated because the slack was taken up by the first person's one foot pull. Now, for completeness sake, assume these two people are now only five feet apart, if either of them pulls one foot of rope separately or together, it doesn't matter as they don't have the ability to take up the excess slack in the rope.

If the humeral head translates superiorly within the Gleno-humeral joint, not only does it compromise the lever arm of the Deltoid but it also weakens its optimal contraction. In some cases, when a person has a large tear of their rotator cuff, the humeral head cannot be centered, and translates and moves up superiorly out of the glenoid and rubs on the acromion. (figure 17) If that person tries to elevate their arm the Deltoid fires but the arm doesn't move because, the Deltoid moment arm is shortened, and the Deltoid cannot contract enough to take 'up the slack.' So even though the Deltoid is working, it cannot do its job.

This re-enforces the importance of the rotator cuff and in particular the supra-spinatus. Not only does the supraspinatus muscle unit aid in elevation of the humerus/arm, its more important role is to keep the humeral head centered within the joint. This deserves repeating; the major role of the Supraspinatous and the muscles of the rotator cuff is to constantly keep the humeral head centered within the glenoid socket. This keeps the larger muscles at their optimal muscle length, keeps their moment arms most efficient and lastly adds dynamic stability to the joint.

When the Deltoid muscle fires to elevate the arm, a major portion of its force vector is straight up. This would drive the humeral head into the acromion, if the rotator cuff did not center the humeral head. This would cause pain and make the contraction relatively ineffective in some cases. Again, the rotator cuff depresses the humeral head, keeping it centered and allows the Deltoid to do its job.

Again, when the Deltoid fires, the Supraspinatus muscle fires at the same time. The Supraspinatus' vector force is as a humeral head depressor. This is key to the action of arm elevation as it keeps the center of rotation nearly constant, and the length and lever arm of the Deltoid most efficient.

It may seem that I have spent an incredibly excessive amount of time on this, but this force action couple is the cornerstone a proper functioning shoulder. When this coupling doesn't work, it can lead to injury and fixing the force couple and rotator cuff function is key to recovery from injury. This will be touched upon multiple times in upcoming sections of the book.

THE ACROMIO-CLAVICULAR JOINT

The Acromio-clavicular joint, also known simply as the AC Joint, is where the scapula, and thereby the arm, skeletally connects to the axial skeleton. On the medial side of the acromion is a joint that articulates with the clavicle. As we travel towards the midline of the body medially, the clavicle connects with the sternum, which connects to the ribs which wrap around the chest and connects to the thoracic vertebrae. It is only through this series of joint connections that the arm is connected to the axial skeleton of the body. (figures 8,18)

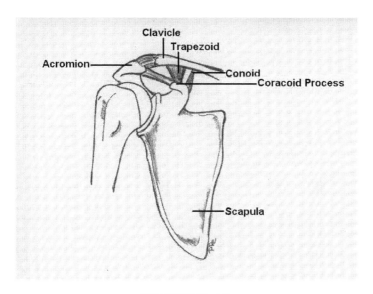

FIGURE 18

The AC joint is surrounded by its capsule, the primary stabilizer of the joint. In addition, the scapula has other connections to the clavicle. On the front of the scapula, is a bony projection to which multiple ligaments and muscles attach. It is called the coracoid process. From the coracoid process originates two ligaments that attach to the clavicle about two centimeters medial to the AC Joint. These ligaments, the conoid and trapezoid, so named for their shape, are secondary stabilizers of the AC Joint as well as secondary connectors of the scapula, and thus the arm, to the axial skeleton. (figure 18)

The clavicle acts as a strut, not only connecting the arm to the body but also keeping it at a set distance from the center of the body and preventing it from collapsing inward and forward. The clavicle keeps the scapula/shoulder retracted back on the chest wall where it is most efficient and least prone to injury. Its function is similar to the strut and control arm on the wheel of a car. The muscles of the scapula that attach the scapula to the spine and chest wall function most efficiently when they are at a certain length. The clavicle keeps the scapula at a fixed distance from the axial skeleton and thereby keeps the scapular muscles at an optimal length. The clavicle also acts as a lever arm for the scapula to rotate on, similar to the discussion about the Deltoid lever arm action on the humerus.

SCAPULO-THORACIC JOINT

The scapula has its own attachment to the axial skeleton, but it is not a direct or bony attachment. It is attached to the axial skeleton and rib cage posteriorly, on the back, by muscles. (figure 19, 20)

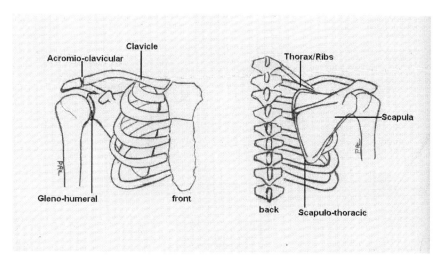

FIGURE 19

The scapula sits on our back and moves across our upper posterior thoracic chest wall. It does not articulate in the usual sense as a true joint with articular cartilage, but it does have contact with the chest wall and moves along its surface. This scapular motion does constitute a significant portion of the motion achieved by the shoulder and in abduction of the arm, can account for upwards of a third of the total elevation achieved, with the larger portion being achieved through the Gleno-humeral joint.

The major muscles that attach the scapula to the chest wall and body are the Pectoralis Major and Serratus Anterior on the anterior surface of the scapula, and the

Rhomboid Major and Minor, the Levator Scapulae, Trapezius and a portion of the Latissimus Dorsi along its posterior and medial boarder. These muscle groups play an important role in stabilizing the shoulder. It is accomplished by setting a stable platform of the scapula in relation to the body, and the rest of the shoulder and arm builds upon it. These muscles play an integral role in posture as well as secondary motion about the shoulder. (figure 20)

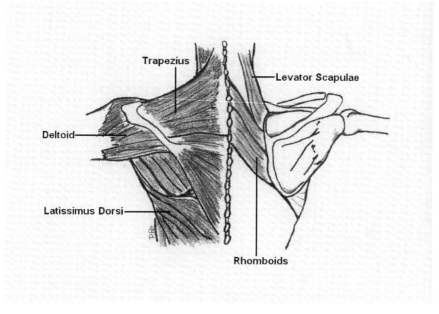

FIGURE 20

So in summary, the shoulder is actually made up of three joints: The AC joint uses the clavicle to connect the scapula to the chest. The clavicle acts like a strut keeping the scapula sitting on our back where it is most efficient. The Scapulo-thoracic joint which is not an articular joint but is where the scapula moves up down forward and backward to allow better arm and hand position. The muscles that attach the scapula to the back stabilize the scapula and set a strong platform for the arm and hand to be used. The third is the Gleno-humeral joint. This is what most people think of when they think of the shoulder. It is a true ball in socket articular joint, and its inherent instability gives it incredible motion.

The rotator cuff muscles, while they do play a role in the motion of the Gleno-humeral joint, their more important roles are their constant centering of the humeral head ball within the glenoid socket. This gives dynamic stabilization to the Gleno-humeral joint. The ligaments and capsule provide the static stabilization. By constantly centering the Gleno-himeral joint, the rotator cuff muscles allow the bigger work horse muscles around the shoulder to do their job by keeping their moment arm at a good distance and their muscle fibers at an appropriate length to allow for full optimal contraction.

INJURY

INTRODUCTION

In this next section we will discuss different common injuries to the shoulder. They will include traumatic and non-traumatic rotator cuff tears, rotator cuff tendonitis, instability, stiffness, arthritis and how daily life plays a major role in both the injury and rehabilitation from injury

ROTATOR CUFF TEARS

Rotator cuff tears can be broken down into traumatic and non-traumatic tears. While all rotator cuff injuries can be traced to some initial form of trauma (whether it be a fall or just raking leaves that might lead to tendonitis that eventually causes tearing), we consider traumatic injuries those tears that are caused by a definitive finite event (e.g. a fall on an outstretched arm, slip on some ice, fall from a ladder, etc.). The mechanism of injury can be simple; the force from the fall loads the arm which in turn loads the rotator cuff. The mechanism may be different. In one scenario, a person falls onto their outstretched arm. That arm braces their body and gets loaded with the force of the fall. That load translates up the arm into the humerus and then the humeral head gets forced into the acromion bone above it. The supraspinatus tendon gets pinched between the two and can tear.

Another mechanism is that with the fall, the arm gets forcefully pulled down or into the body or across it. In response, the rotator cuff contracts to stabilize the joint, and the two forces acting in opposite directions overload the rotator cuff tendon and it tears. (figure 21).

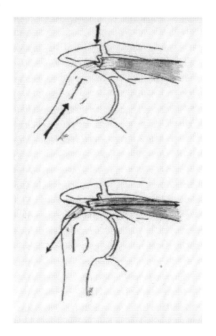

FIGURE 21

An additional example is if we slip. Instinctively, we throw our arms up in the air to balance our selves.

The sudden uncontrolled, unbalanced elevation and muscle contraction, can overload the tendon and cause it to tear.

In these scenarios, a specific event caused the tear. What usually follows is a period of pain. The shoulder initially swells as do the muscles and tendons about it. It may stiffen up, but as the stiffness slowly resolves so does the pain. During that period of time that the muscles and tendons are swollen, they do not function properly. The torn muscle tendon unit isn't functioning but neither are the intact swollen ones. That is because a swollen muscle cannot function appropriately and this leads to further pain and dysfunction. This is the key problem with rotator cuff tendonitis that will be expanded upon later. During this phase the whole shoulder isn't functioning appropriately and that not only leads to pain and the inability to properly assess the full extent of the injury, but it can also lead to more damage. As the swelling dissipates and the other intact muscle-tendon units recover and function, if the tear is small enough, the other intact tendons can compensate for the torn part by the force couple load sharing described earlier in the rotator cuff section. In low demand situations this person with a torn rotator cuff can continue to function. The problem that can occur in this situation is that in time, this tear can, and usually does get bigger.

Just like a small tear in the cloth of a flag, that small tear, as it sees continued force moving in the wind, will continue to tear and tear. And in the case of the shoulder, a small tear may not initially be very painful, but continued use can cause the tear to get bigger. Not only are larger tears more difficult to repair and heal, but as a tear becomes more chronic, the cuff tendon and muscle lose its elasticity, and may not be able to be stretched back into position. Think of it this way. If you tear a tendon, the muscle attached to it contracts and pulls that tendon away from where it normally attached. In this contracted postion, the muscle scars in and atrophies. Sometimes, if you try to repair these, the amount of scar and atrophy that has occurred make it impossible for you to pull it out to length and reattach it back. Also, at times the tendon is so weakened and atrophied that it won't hold the suture needed to fix it. That is why we often recommend fixing even small tears in the healthy and active patient.

Now, if you have a tear that is big enough that strengthening your other intact rotator cuff muscles cannot compensate for, you end up with a bigger problem. The most commonly torn rotator cuff tendon is the Supraspinatous. The Supraspinatous is on top of the humeral head and its most important function is to depress the humeral head so that when the Deltoid fires to initiate arm elevation, the humeral head and thereby center of rotation remains centered within the glenoid socket. If the Supraspinatous cannot depress the humeral head and center it when the Deltoid fires, the humeral head rises up superiorly out of the glenoid socket. A couple of things happen next. First, the humeral head can then hit and rub on the undersurface of the acromion. This causes pain and can start to wear away the articular cartilage where contact is made. It is possible that after it hits the acromion, the Deltoid may have sufficient force to continue to elevate the arm by levering/wedging the humeral head up into the under surface of the acromion. (figure 17)

But as this continues, a couple of things happen.

First, the rotator cuff tear gets bigger. This results in the humeral head superiorly translating and chronically rubbing on the acromion. Next, this superior postion and subluxation causes abnormal mechanics at the normal glenoid socket and now the patient develops arthritis there. Lastly, both situations become so great that the tear is so big that the Deltoid cannot elevate the arm, and on top of that, the patient has significant wear of the cartilage and arthritis pain. Essentially they are left with a chronically painful shoulder that they cannot lift or use. The tendon tear is so large, contracted and scarred in, that the tear is not repairable. This is a problem with no easy solution.

For these reasons and more, a torn rotator cuff tendon in the active, healthy person should be repaired.

In discussing rotator cuff tears one must also consider atraumatic tears. An atraumatic tear is a tear that occurs without a discreet defined event or no specific trauma. They are usually a result of chronic rotator cuff tendonitis which weakens the tendon. Also as we age, our tendons weaken due to its decrease in flexibility and hydration. They occur as a result of chronic rubbing of the tendon on the undersurface of the acromion. If someone has a bone spur on the under surface of the acromion, this further can cause excess rubbing and swelling.

The chronically swollen tendon leads to cell death in that tendon and eventual structural failure and a tear. The rotator cuff has a tenuous blood supply that brings nutrients to the living cells within the tendon. These cells constantly repair and keep the tendon alive. If the tendon is chronically swollen, it pinches off and chokes off the blood supply to the cells in the tendon. These cells function poorly and eventually can die. The tendon cannot maintain or repair itself and eventually structural failure and a tear occurs. When you have chronic rubbing of the tendon on the acromion, eventually the tendon fails by direct rubbing. These ideas will be further discussed in the next section on rotator cuff tendonitis.

ROTATOR CUFF TENDONITIS

Rotator Cuff Tendonitis can be traumatic, attritional or atraumatic (without trauma). One can say that all damage to the rotator cuff is traumatic, but we will define that traumatic tendonitis is a result of a finite injury; like raking the leaves, lifting a heavy suitcase or overdoing it at the gym. These types of finite injuries, like the rotator cuff tears, can cause a forceful stretch of the rotator cuff or a direct blow, which pinches the cuff under the acromion. Either way, the result is micro damage to the tendon and swelling. (figure 22)

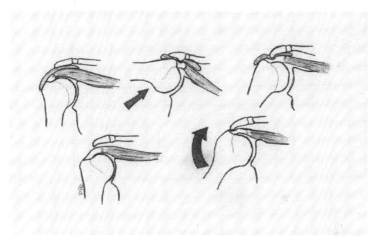

FIGURE 22

This swelling of the tendon causes alteration of function, and begins a cycle of repetitive injury and cell death.

A swollen tendon muscle unit does not function well. The normal elasticity of the tendon decreases as does the contractility of the muscle. This results in a unit that does not work even though it is intact. In the case of a swollen Supraspinatous, when you want to elevate your arm and the Deltoid fires, the intact Supraspinatous does not function appropriately and does not depress the humeral head. As a result, the humeral head subluxes superiorly and hits/rubs against the acromion leading to further injury, swelling and dysfunction. This is what we call the cycle of repetitive injury; A swollen muscle tendon unit does not function. Then when you try to raise your arm the Deltoid pulls the humeral head up and the Supraspinatous tendon rubs on the undersurface of the acromion. This causes more trauma to the tendon which makes it more swollen, more injured and even less likely to function correctly which reinforces the injury cycle.

In the uninjured shoulder when you elevate the arm and the Deltoid fires and the Supraspinatous fires concomitantly, it glides unharmed in that finite space. However, if the Supraspinatous tendon is swollen to let's say twice its normal size, (figure 23) it has now filled that finite space and is now chronically rubbing up against the undersurface of the acromion, causing more pain, more direct trauma, and more swelling thereby reinforcing the cycle and leading to a chronic problem. This chronic swelling can lead to cell death and ultimate tendon failure.

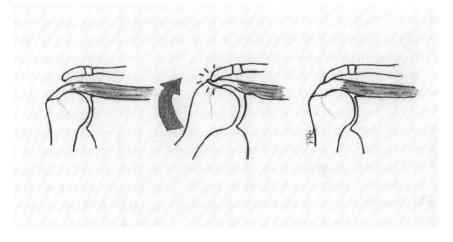

FIGURE 23

To understand this phenomenon better, let's review some basic information. Injury to the rotator cuff tendon, or any tendon for that matter, is generically called tendinopathy. Terms more commonly used is tendinitis and tendinosis. Tendinosis represents chronic, possibly permanent damage to the tendon beyond tendonitis.

In tendinitis there is a stretching and injury to the fibroblasts in the tendon which leads to inflammatory mediators and swelling of the tendon. This usually occurs within the first few weeks of the injury. If you can get rid of the swelling, and remove or resolve the injury, the tendon can recover quickly. However, if you have continued injury and swelling after a couple of months, biopsies will show tendinosis. In tendinosis you rarely see inflammatory cells. There is degeneration of the tendon, a loss of the tightly bundled collagen formation and a beginning of fibrosis and scarring of the tendon. If you look at the tendon grossly, the increased size or thickness is less due to swelling but more due to the degenerative fibrosis. It is harder to heal from tendinosis, which is a more permanent change. The use of anti-inflammatory medications like ibuprofen and steroids are unlikely to work because it is no longer a problem with inflammation.

Now if tendinosis continues and more degeneration and fibrosis continues, then the tendon becomes weaker and can fail under lighter loads. In addition, in both tendonitis and tendinosis, the swelling and thickening of fibrosis can cause compression to the blood vessels supplying the tendon, poor oxygenation (anoxia), further injury and cell death. The reason this happens is multifactorial. First we have to understand that the undersurface of the rotator cuff is what is known as a watershed area. That is, it has a poor vascular blood supply that is at the very end of the vascular channels, and is at risk for low flow anoxia (not enough oxygen being delivered).

The injury of a tendon being pinched under the acromion causes more anoxia to the underside of the tendon than to the side actually rubbing against it. In addition, swelling of the tendon will constrict the blood flow to the tendon further causing anoxia and more extensive permanent damage. Finally, in response to this, there is a revascularization that occurs in tendinosis. However, this new formation of blood vessels within the tendon to aid in healing actually weakens the tendon by resorption. So the body in trying to heal itself, brings in new blood vessels that structurally weaken the tendon. If the tendon recovers, then the strength can return to normal, but if you continue to injure the tendon during this process, it can fail and tear more easily. (figure 24)

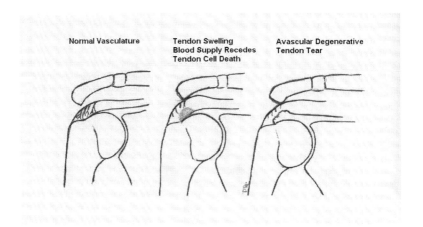

FIGURE 24

Now we can see that a simple injury can lead to swelling, repetitive injury, cell death and ultimate tendon failure without a specific traumatic injury. That being noted, it further shows the importance of avoiding injury, or if you can't avoid injury, the importance of getting rid of the swelling as fast as possible, and breaking the cycle of repetitive injury. This will be discussed later in the section on healing and preventing injury.

So in traumatic rotator cuff tendonitis, our ability to recover from that injury will define whether we return to our normal state of shoulder health, or fall into the cycle of repetitive injury.

Atraumatic, or non-traumatic tendonitis is not caused by a finite injury, but rather a continued cycle of small injuries. So the term non-traumatic is in reality a misnomer, but is used because patients do not have a single event causing it. I like to call these micro-repetitive traumas. Either the tendon rubbing on the acromion or repetitive overloading of the tendon which each can cause injury and swelling.

Most of these are caused by repetitive work, sports or exercises with poor mechanics. Most of us live our lives in what I call 'A position of Potential Injury.' We are primed to injure ourselves. In the balance between protected body posture and mechanics, and injured position, we live tilted toward the injured position. That is, we carry ourselves with such poor posture and go about our lives functioning and performing tasks with such poor mechanics that we live on the verge of constant injury. This is due to a number of factors.

First is our posture, both axial and scapular. In particular reference to the axial spine, most of us have acquired a hunched forward upper back. This is medically called a kyphotic upper thoracic alignment to our spine in the sagital plane. (figure 25)

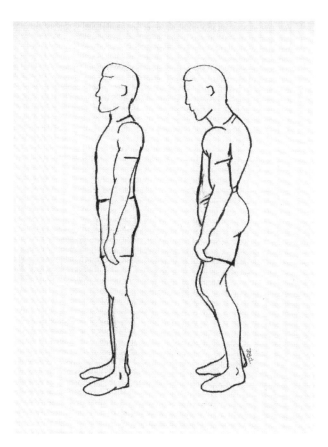

FIGURE 25

This is caused by tightness in our hip flexors and anterior chest musculature among other factors. We have developed this in response to a sitting lifestyle in work, leisure, and driving. Also mechanical laborers, although strong, are stronger in their anterior chest musculature and weaker in their backs. This kyphotic position humps our spine back posteriorly and our scapulas/shoulders roll/rotate anteriorly or forward. (figures 25, 26)

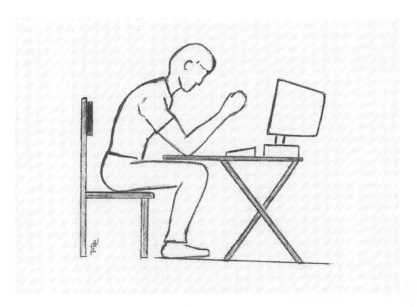

FIGURE 26

As I like to say to my patients, "We all live our lives in front of ourselves." Most everything we do is accomplished with us looking forward and using our limbs in front of us. This reinforces this poor posture. Our anterior chest muscles are overused, tighten up and pull our shoulder blades (scapulas) forward.

In fact, this problem is further worsened by people's best intentions. That is, when we decide after years of inactivity to get back in shape, many of us choose to lift weights and among the most popular is the bench press. Out of all of the upper body exercises we do, it is the one that most of us can lift the largest amount of weight so that makes us feel good. We get that nice burn, that pumped feeling and we can see results of the workout more quickly than other groups. For the same amount of time and effort these muscles get stronger quicker and to a greater degree than our back musculature. Sounds great but the problem is that it worsens our problem by rotating and rolling our shoulders forward setting us up for injury if our eager exercise did not already do so.

How this occurs goes back to our initial anatomy lesson where we described the scapular morphology and its acromial relationship with the rotator cuff tendon below it. There exists a limited amount of space between the two. With the scapula in its correct position, when we elevate our arm not only are the muscular moment arms more efficient as we described, but the humeral head can rotate more smoothly and if it does hit any structure above it, it is more likely to be soft tissue.

However, if we have poor posture and our scapula is rolled forward (this is called protracted), the acromial roof closes over the top of the humeral head. (figure 27)

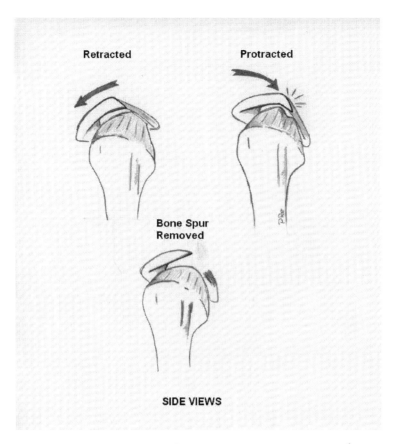

Retracted　　　　　Protracted

Bone Spur
Removed

SIDE VIEWS

FIGURE 27

In this position, when we elevate our arm, the rotator cuff tendon is more likely to hit and rub against the acromion bone instead of soft tissue. Now if there is a bone spur on the undersurface of the acromion, the rubbing and pinching is more severe. This phenomenon sets us up for repeated injury over time which can cause the cycle of repetitive injury that we previously talked about.

An unstable shoulder, be it due to a torn capsule, a patulous capsule or weak rotator cuff musculature, causes the shoulder to move and sublux inappropriately within its joint. This causes damage by direct trauma to the tendons around it or indirectly by allowing the tendons to hit and rub against structure around it including the acromion and coracoid process. Again, this is not a finite traumatic event, but a repetitive and cumulative micro trauma.

Last, evolution plays a part in our upright posture. We have developed an anatomical alignment in which our scapula is supposed to sit posteriorly on our back with our arms by our side.

In this position, we have a limited range of motion; in particular let's focus on external rotation, rotating our arms outward. The average person can externally rotate their arms 60 degrees with their arms by their sides. This is more than sufficient to achieve our daily tasks of living. Now if over time we assume a more anterior, protracted scapular/shoulder position, we lose resultant external rotation.

Try it; sitting upright with your arm by your side,

and your elbow bent to 90 degrees. In this position externally rotate as much as you can and see how much you have achieved. Now keeping your arm there, roll and protract your shoulders forward and hunch your upper back. Now notice the inward resultant rotation of your arm. While the external rotation of the arm in relation to the scapula may not have changed, since the scapula is now more internally rotated, we effectively lost some external functional motion. (figure 28) This sets us up for injury if in that poor postured position, we force our arms to get that extra external rotation. This injury is caused by overuse, and over stretch. In addition, in a position of poor scapular posture, our muscles now have to work in a plane outside their optimal position.

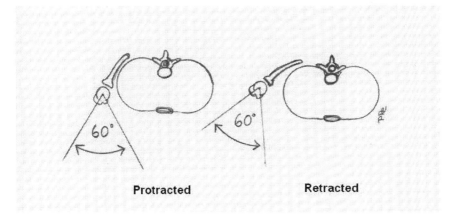

FIGURE 28

Whether traumatic, non-traumatic or repetitive micro traumatic, the essentials of treatment for rotator cuff tendonitis is the same. Decrease and eliminate swelling as quickly as possible, obtain and maintain correct scapular posture and mechanics, and obtain and maintain the strength and functionality of the injured as well as uninjured tendon-muscle units.

ADHESIVE CAPSULITIS
FROZEN SHOULDER

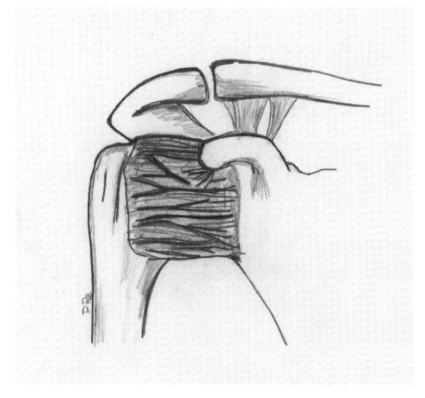

FIGURE 29

One of the more perplexing and most painful conditions of the shoulder is "Frozen Shoulder." It is a condition in which the shoulder's motion is extremely limited and even more painful. Frozen shoulder is also known as Adhesive Capsulitis but frozen shoulder is more commonly used and relates to the three phases that people use to describe the condition. First is the 'freezing phase,' when the shoulder becomes progressively more stiff. Next is the 'frozen phase,' when the shoulder has limited or no motion. Last is the 'thawing phase,' when the motion gradually returns. Each phase usually lasts about 4-6 months, however in some patients, full resolution can take two to three years.

A frozen shoulder usually occurs between the ages of 40 to 65 and is more common in women. It affects about 3-5% of the general population and up to 20% of diabetics. Although rarely occurring in both shoulders at the same time, 40% of the time patients will experience it in their other shoulder at some point. Nobody truly knows nor understands why it happens, but there exists a definite correlation with other disease processes including diabetes, stroke, and heart disease. There may be some autoimmune component as well as a correlation with menopause.

We really do not know why it occurs, or why some people are more prone to it. When patients ask me why I think it occurs, I tell them that I believe it is an abnormal healing response to an injury that had occurred prior to their shoulder freezing. Most patients present only once they have lost a significant amount of motion. That is because they didn't notice their gradual loss of motion. The reason they didn't notice it is because we rarely use the limits of our motion and when we do experience minor limits, we can turn our body and use our scapula to compensate. Because of that, we don't notice the early loss of motion and patients can present to the office three months after the process had already begun without their noticing. So to that end, a patient could have had an injury for 3-4 months prior to them noticing a limitation.

Once I explain that progression to them, in a significant number of cases, patients often recall an injury such as falling on the ice, skiing, lifting a suitcase out of an overhead bin or similar event. They had a minor injury that caused some inflammation for a week or so and gradually improved, but as their pain resolved and they forgot the injury, their shoulder was slowly stiffening up on them. Months later it is so stiff that it causes pain with daily activity and while sleeping.

The reason why a frozen shoulder is so painful is based on a couple of factors. First, the actual stiffness and irritation to the shoulder causes pain. But, if you have a stiff shoulder and you move it, a couple of things happen. First, stretching the shoulder past the amount the stiff capsule allows causes direct trauma to that already stiff painful reactive capsule. Second, in the uninjured shoulder, as you rotate your shoulder externally or outwards, the capsule allows the motion and stretches a little and the humeral head remains centered within the glenoid socket. When you have a stiff frozen shoulder, when you rotate your shoulder out, instead of it externally rotating outwardly and remaining centered, it coils superiorly because the stiff capsule stops the rotation and forces the humeral head upwards, out of center and the rotator cuff and bursa get pinched under the roof of the acromion.

The last significant source of pain comes from the compensatory actions of the shoulder. Since the desired motion cannot be achieved through the Gleno-humeral joint, you compensate for it by using your Scapulo-thoracic joint. Meaning that the scapula has to move abnormally on your back. This causes pain in the stabilizing muscles that connect the scapula to the spine, neck and axial skeleton. This occurs because they get stretched abnormally and since they are being used in a way they were not designed, causes more pain and spasms.

Treatment for frozen shoulder is rarely successful during the freezing phase. In fact, formal physical therapy can cause more pain and more scaring by irritating an already reactive shoulder. The goal of treatment during the 'freezing phase' is to decrease the inflammatory reactive process and limit motion loss. Basically we want to shorten the 'freezing phase'. To do this we use anti-inflammatory medications including non-steroidals and corticosteroids as needed. We do encourage a gentle home stretching program to stop or slow down the progressive loss of motion. Once we are out of the 'freezing phase' and into the 'frozen phase,' is when we get more aggressive. This includes either a more aggressive home program of stretching or a formalized therapy program and the continued use of anti-inflammatory medication as needed. In some cases, we need to inject the corticosteroids into the shoulder bursa as well as directly into the joint, in order to get the medicine on both sides of the capsule. This is accomplished using an ultrasound machine, which shows us the anatomy so we can place the needle in the exact correct position. With guided support, most patients do get better with time. In my practice, I have also found that patients who are prone to anxiety and stress, experience a more significant and refractory form of this disease. In these patients I sometimes include prescription medication for anxiety, stress management and nerve blocks as needed. In more complicated cases, adhesive capsulitis may be part of a more involved process called RSD (Reflex Sympathetic Dystrophy) - also referred to as Complex Regional Pain Syndrome. In these rare cases, the nerves around the shoulder are in a hyper-sensitive state and they get into a complex reflex cycle of pain that bypasses any signal sent back to the brain and self-reinforces itself. These cases are particularly painful and difficult to treat, and are treated with consultation with neurologists, use of medications that were originally used to treat seizures, and the use of nerve blocks.

Acupuncture can also play a significant role in pain reduction. While I do not have the expertise or experience to comment on how acupuncture can or cannot affect whole body health or disease processes, it is clear, that in my practice acupuncture can help decrease pain by blocking or breaking pain cycles and relieving muscles spasms. I often refer my patients with refractory pain to a neurologist with a sub specialty in acupuncture, or a licensed acupuncturist and have been pleased with results.

As mentioned earlier, most people do get better. And by most I mean nearly everyone if they are able to manage the pain and give it time. I tell my patients that if your pain is controlled and you are able to function in your daily activities of life without notable pain or limitations, and are able to sleep at night, then you can continue to wait as the body heals over time. Unfortunately, there are some patients who do not improve, have severe unresolving pain that affects their sleep, work and function during simple activities of daily living. These patients are candidates to have a procedure or procedures performed (e.g. a manipulation under anesthesia or an arthroscopic procedure to remove the adhesions and scar, loosen the capsule and remove any offending component to the shoulder including a bone spur if present).

These procedures are very successful if needed and are done as a day procedure arthroscopically (using small incisions, mini arthroscopes and micro-instrumentation). During the procedure, adhesions and scar is removed both from the inside and outside of the joint. The stiff capsule is loosened and any bone spur that is irritating the shoulder is removed. Lastly, the shoulder is gently stretched (manipulated) to ensure full motion is achieved. Immediately after the surgery patients note that their pain they were previously experiencing is gone and that say that they are just dealing with post-operative recovery pain. Usually by four weeks after the surgery, they feel better than they did before the procedure and by 2-3 months they have near full function.

While we can't control some of the risk factors that make us more prone to a frozen shoulder, we can lessen our likelihood of suffering from a frozen shoulder by increasing our flexibly, and having good mechanics with a well-balanced and strengthened shoulder. Sound familiar?

SHOULDER INSTABILITY

Instability of the shoulder can be broken down into two major types; traumatic and non-traumatic.

As the name implies, traumatic instability is the result of a force acting upon the shoulder leading to the humeral head subluxating or dislocating out of the socket of the glenoid. The cross sectional anatomy of the Gleno-humeral joint is similar to a golf ball sitting on a golf tee and is inherently unstable. The labral cartilage that surrounds the lip of the glenoid, 'deepens the socket of the glenoid,' adding some more stability by increasing the surface area of the glenoid and covering more of the humeral head. (figure 9)

The remainder of the static stability is made up by the Gleno-humeral ligaments that cradle the humeral head superiorly, inferiorly and posteriorly. When the arm is abducted and externally rotated, the anterior middle and inferior Gleno-humeral ligaments coil and tighten to further provide a buttress to anterior translation forces as commonly seen in throwing.

The traumatic instability can either be a repetitive

micro trauma or a finite event that is significant enough to tear the anterior or posterior capsulop-labral stabilizing complex or rarely fracture the lip of the genoid, breaking off a piece of bone with the capsule and labrum attached.

An excellent example of repetitive micro trauma is seen in throwers, especially pitchers. Over the years, the repetitive stress of throwing and placing abnormally high amounts of load to the abducted externally rotated arm can cause the anterior stabilizing ligaments to stretch out and loosen.

If the pitcher has poor mechanics, and a weak rotator cuff, the humeral head subluxes anteriorly out of the glenoid socket and the undersurface of the rotator cuff rubs against the posterior lip of the glenoid posteriorly causing tendonitis and possible partial tearing. This is known as posterior internal glenoid impingement. (figure 30)

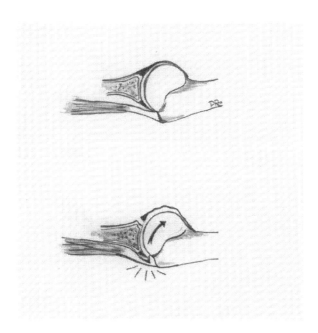

FIGURE 30

The best treatment for this is avoiding the injury by once again having the appropriate mechanics, form and rotator cuff strength. If it does occur, then usually a course of anti-inflamatories and rehabilitation can cure the problem. While the program does include a generalized strengthening and stretching program of the rotator cuff, it generally focuses on strengthening of the anterior shoulder stabilizers and stretching of the posterior capsule. Only in the rare case is it necessary to perform surgery in which the rotator cuff may be repaired and the anterior capsule-labral complex tightened. Once the anterior capsule is tightened, the humeral head no longer slides forward and the rotator cuff no longer pinches on the glenoid.

Finite event occurrences are usually either anterior or posterior dislocations. Anterior dislocations are much more common than posterior for a couple of reasons. Most sports and physical tasks put our shoulder in a position that places our anterior shoulder structures at risk for injury. In addition, our posterior shoulder and rotator cuff musculature are much more robust and are stronger than the anterior. This fact is believed to provide more dynamic stability to the posterior shoulder.

Because of this muscular distribution, when a patient does present with a posterior dislocation of the Gleno-humeral shoulder joint, seizure and electrocution are among the leading likely causes. In both of these causes, there occurs such a significant powerful muscular contraction that the posterior muscles, being stronger, overpower the anterior muscles and pull the humeral head posteriorly out of the glenoid socket. So when evaluating a person with a posterior dislocation, one must rule out a seizure or electrocution.

Once reduced, posterior dislocations are quite stable

for the reasons we have previously listed and can be rehabilitated well because of the potential of strong dynamic muscle recruitment. It is rare that a posterior dislocation needs to be repaired.

The converse is true for anterior dislocations. Once a traumatic dislocation occurs anteriorly, the recurrence rate is inversely proportional to the age of the patient at first dislocation, proportionally related to the number of times dislocated, and related to the type of activity or sport the patient wants to return to. Classically, first time anterior dislocations were treated non-operatively with a course of immobilization followed by rehabilitation to strengthen the anterior musculature. Recent studies suggest that immobilization of the arm in slight external rotation may cause better apposition of the torn anterior structures, however it has not been proven to make a definitive difference. Surgical stabilization was reserved for those patients who had dislocated twice within one year or more than three times total. However, these more recent studies are also suggesting more aggressive surgical treatment for first time dislocators who have injured their dominant side and participate in overhead sports or repetitive activity. In fact, for active patients younger than 35 who dislocate their shoulder, their risk of dislocating their shoulder again is more than 50%. Either way, the importance of mechanics, posture and rotator cuff strengthening is important in a rehabilitation program either post-injury or post-operatively.

The last type of traumatic dislocations that I would like to mention are the cases in which either the rotator cuff also tears or the edge lip of the glenoid breaks off or is fractured. Having the rotator cuff also tear with a shoulder dislocation, is more common in patients older than 45, and when this occurs, a repair of the cuff and torn capsule-labral complex is necessary because they are significantly more unstable than the simple dislocations. This is due to the fact that our shoulder is a closed system. If the humeral head is distracted or moved away from the glenoid, a negative suction pressure develops which gives it more stability. Think of a cork in a wine bottle. As you pull out the cork, it is more difficult because it is a closed system and a negative pressure develops. That is why you hear the pop when the cork is finally removed. If you drill a hole in the bottle before you remove the cork, it is incredibly easier. You have 'opened up the system.' In the shoulder, if you have a torn rotator cuff, in addition to losing the dynamic stabilization function of the cuff, the hole in the tendon makes the shoulder an open system, you lose that negative pressure dynamic and the shoulder is inherently more unstable.

In the case where the glenoid lip is fractured, in the large majority of cases, surgical repair is also warranted. This can be understood by returning to that cross sectional view of the Gleno-humeral joint and relating it to a golf ball on a golf tee. Now imagine taking that golf tee and breaking off the edge of it. (Figure 31)

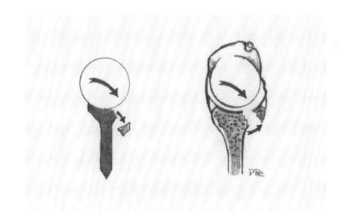

FIGURE 31

This would dramatically increase the instability of

the situation and cause the golf ball to fall off. The same is true with the glenoid; once more than 15% or so is broken off and displaced, the inherent stability of the shoulder is greatly decreased because in addition to losing the stabilizing effects of the torn labrum and capsule, the surface area of the glenoid is now decreased and the socket has become more shallow. The instability of the shoulder has increased, as has a higher probability of recurrent dislocations, damage and limitations to that shoulder. For these reasons, if the glenoid lip is significantly broken and displaced, surgical repair is warranted.

Once again, in both cases, appropriate mechanics, posture and strengthening of the rotator cuff musculature is invaluable for full and appropriate recovery.

ARTHRITIS

Arthritis is the wear/breakdown of articular cartilage and it occurs for many reasons. Commonly, people think that arthritis is when the joint space on X-ray is no longer visible, and boney thickening (sclerosis) and spurs (osteophytes) are formed. While these are later manifestation of arthritis, arthritis begins with the simple fissuring and breakdown of articular cartilage that doesn't even show up on x-rays. There are many causes of arthritis, but the two major forms are inflammatory and osteoarthritis. In inflammatory arthritis, the patient's immune system attacks its own tissue including the lining of joints causing swelling, pain and eventual joint destruction. Rheumatoid Arthritis is a form of inflammatory arthritis. In osteoarthritis, there are two major forms; traumatic and degenerative. In traumatic osteoarthritis, there is a specific injury that acts upon the articular cartilage that causes breakdown of the normal surface. This leads to abnormal loading characteristics and progressive wear and degeneration. In degenerative arthritis, also called wear and tear arthritis, as we age, the cartilage breaks down. This is due to many factors. Chief among those factors is that as we age, the ability of our cartilage to hold fluid and remain hydrated decreases. This is due to the progressive degeneration of the cartilage's scaffold building structures known as proteoglycans. As this happens, the cartilage loses its ability to hold water and becomes more brittle. As the cartilage becomes less hydrated it becomes more brittle and breaks down.

In either form, it is quite painful. Shoulder arthritis is not as common as knee or hip arthritis as the hip and knee are weight bearing joints and see more load and forces acting upon them. Even when a patient does have significant shoulder arthritis, it still may not be that limiting because the shoulder is not a weight bearing joint. Also, patients can compensate for their shoulder's limitation by using their other arm/shoulder, or altering their mechanics.

In the cases in which patients do have symptomatic shoulder arthritis, the pain is multifactorial. The most obvious source of pain comes from the wearing away of the joint and articular cartilage. A secondary source of pain originates from a secondary inflammation that accompanies the degeneration as well as joint swelling. This causes the resultant surrounding joint capsule and rotator cuff to swell as well. In the case of the rotator cuff, what results is a tendonitis and the symptoms and problems associated with that. When the capsule swells, it gets stiffer and scarred and results in a stiff painful shoulder and the problems associated with an adhesive capsulitis or frozen shoulder. In the case of shoulder arthritis, the symptoms can be far worse. The stiff capsule causes increased joint reactive forces and increased shear and load onto an already damaged articular surface and this further accelerates the arthritic process.

Treatment of shoulder arthritis is first focused on addressing the primary cause and treating that when possible. The secondary treatment plans focus on a couple of things. First is decreasing the inflammation in the joint. This can be addressed with medicines such as anti-inflammatories as well as corticosteroids, and those directed at controlling inflammatory arthritis. Other ways to decrease inflammation is to treat the tendonitis with a rehabilitation protocol that focuses once again on form, posture and mechanics. However, in these cases a significant goal and purpose of therapy is to increase range of motion of the shoulder. If you can stretch out the shoulder's joint capsule you increase the shoulder's range of motion and thereby decrease the shear joint reactive forces that the arthritic articular cartilage experiences. By doing so, you can thereby decrease the pain you experience and improve your function.

This is accomplished through a series of stretching exercises that stretch out the joint capsule resulting in an increased range of motion and decreased joint reactive forces. In some cases, arthroscopic surgery is used to smooth out joint surfaces, remove scar, loosen the joint capsule, remove loose bodies within the joint, remove bone spurs and treat the tendonitis. If these programs fail and the patient is significantly limited in their daily activities, then a joint replacement surgery may be appropriate.

In any case, capsular pliability, shoulder posture, mechanics and strength play an important role in the pathology and treatment of arthritis of the shoulder and post-surgical rehabilitation if indicated.

LIFE, LIVING AND POSTURE

So, how does simply living life cause shoulder injuries? I mean, if we are not particularly active, participate in sports or strenuous activities, why is it that we are so prone to shoulder injuries. The complex answer is addressed in the next section on the evolution of the shoulder, but the simple answer is: we are not built to live the life we lead, or more appropriately, we don't live life the way we were designed.

Over years of evolution and shoulder development, for many reasons, our shoulders work best, and most efficiently with our scapulas retracted posteriorly and downward on our back. In this position, we are able to achieve the maximum amount of motion of our shoulder and our muscles are in the correct position to work efficiently and with potential of maximum force. All those years growing up, when people told you to sit up and not slouch, they were correct as that slouched position places you at risk for injury. I tell my patients that in that slouched position your body is 'primed' for injury. That the slightest amount of abnormal load or tweak can set off a cascade of injury. The correct positions of our scapulas are with our spine upright and imagining that you are holding an orange between your scapulas. For some people it may be a golf ball, a grapefruit or even a softball, but you get the idea.

The problem is that the life we lead places our body

in the exact opposite position. We as humans evolved as nomadic hunters-gatherers over hundreds of thousands of years. Our bodies were designed and evolved for a life where we would stand and run to hunt, gather foods, and then sit to eat, then lay down and rest.

About 10,000 years ago this dramatically changed with our success in farming. Our intellect and skills with tools made us quite efficient and successful at farming, and our nomadic lives slowly disappeared as we settled down, and developed towns and societies. Over the past couple of hundred years, life has even more dramatically and rapidly changed with the development of the service sector, white collar jobs, transportation and a sedentary lifestyle. Now most of our life is spent sitting at a desk and in front of a computer. The next major portion of our conscious life is spent sitting in a car or train commuting and the next major portion is sitting to eat. This lifestyle lends itself to a hunched and slouched axial spine, rolled forward and hunched shoulders and weakened back musculature. We live our lives in front of us, further reinforcing this poor posture. The only time we work our back muscles or exercise our posture, are the rare occasion that we take to exercise and take care of ourselves. Even then, people rarely exercise the muscles that would help to correct our poor, potentially damaging posture. Instead we mostly focus on our pectoralis, biceps, quadriceps and other anterior musculature which further worsens our posture.

This slouched; rolled forward posture places us at risk for all the injuries we discussed before. Sure we can live most of our lives uninjured, however this poor posture has us primed for an injury once we lift something a little too heavy, rake leaves one weekend, reach behind us in the car to grab something or some other seemingly innocuous activity.

Over millions of years our shoulders slowly evolved and developed to become more efficient and successful in the world and environment we lived. Then, over the past few hundred years, we have dramatically altered our world and environment and our shoulders are no longer optimally designed for use in it. These relatively rapid changes have other huge health implications for the rest of our bodies from a mechanical standpoint. They impact our diet, and contribute to cardiac and renal diseases.

With regard to the shoulder, because of this body/environment mismatch, we are always at risk for injury and a few simple stretches, exercises and posture retraining can minimize that risk.

In the next section on evolution of the shoulder, this idea will be further examined in depth.

EVOLUTION OF THE SHOULDER

The evolution of our shoulder is interesting and complicated. I find it incredibly fascinating and insightful in further unlocking injury patterns and prevention.

Now, I won't start billions of years ago with the formation of the earth, the primordial broth and the source of energy that started it all, rather our journey will begin a few short 15 million years ago when our upright posture branch took a turn away from the other mammals we descended from. I start here because it is this branch that has made us so successful. While other mammals developed forelimbs to improve locomotion, we developed forelimbs for function and agility.

Let us focus on our four 'legged' cousins. Having four legs is particularly useful for a number of reasons including: stability in running and climbing and speed. In regard to speed, certain animals (the Gazelles being herbivores (plant eaters) and the Cheetahs being carnivores (meat eaters)) use this speed for different purposes. Cheetahs have used this increased speed to improve their success in hunting their prey. In the case of their prey, the gazelle, they have used their speed to run away and survive. Another example of the benefit of four limbs used for ambulation is seen in mountain climbers such as the ram or mountain goat. These animals use their four-legged stance to aid in stability in the steep mountainous environment they inhabit. In some cases, they have developed shorter legs that lower their center of gravity which makes them more stable. So these animals have developed their four-legged stance and ambulation to a benefit; speed, agility and stability.

Taking a closer look at the shoulder of two good examples of successful four 'legged' mammals, the horse and dog, we notice some distinct features as compared to humans. Let's focus on the scapulas.

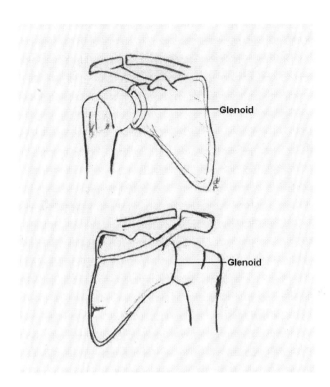

FIGURE 32

Taking a look at the human scapula and in particular the glenoid, we see that it functions in a vertical plane and is rather shallow (figure 32). As we discussed before, this allows for a greater range of motion and particular non-weight bearing function. When we look at the scapula and glenoid of the horse and dog, we see something quite different. (figure 33) In regard to the scapula, we first see it is more oblong shaped and that the scapular spine is oriented more vertically. Next we see that the glenoid plane is more horizontal and more concave, that is, it has more of a 'socket' shape.

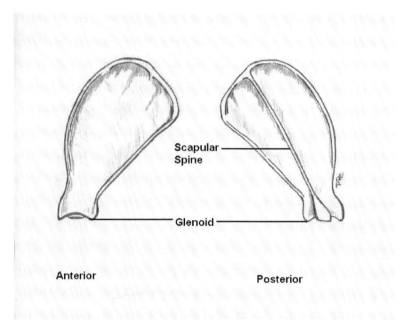

FIGURE 33

This gives more stability to the joint, but less range of motion. While the result is less range of motion, this lost motion isn't needed because the function for this limb is ambulation and speed. It is not the specialized complicated motion and movement that we as human benefit from.

We also see that the scapula, instead of being on the back/dorsal aspect of the thoracic torso (figure 20), is in the more primitive position of remaining on the side of the chest wall. (figure 34) Once again lending itself for a limb well suited for ambulation and stability during ambulation. Speed and four limbed stable ambulation is so essential to dogs and horses that the scapula itself has quite limited motion. To further drive this point home, the dog and horse shoulder unit is so specialized for ambulation, that not only is the scapula on the side of the chest, not only is the glenoid socket more concave, but they do not have a clavicle. In fact, if you examine the shoulder of mammals that specialize in swimming (ie. the whale) or running or grazing, they all have no clavicle. The horse and the dog have no need for a clavicle because their scapula has such a limited range of motion and is stabilized to the chest wall with incredibly strong muscles.

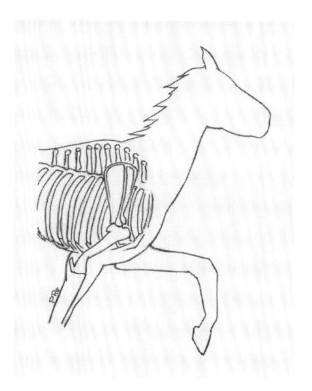

FIGURE 34

So in the case of four legged animals, such as the horse and dog, we see that they have no clavicles, the scapula is on the side of their chest, and the glenoid is facing downward and more concave. These are all adaptations to aid in speed and stability.

If we look at primates who took a turn off our branch, we see that they too have differences in their shoulders as compared to humans.

First starting off with tree monkeys, if we look at their scapula, it is more oblong and the scapula spine, instead of being nearly horizontal like in humans, has more of an oblique upward orientation. In addition, their glenoids don't exist nor function in a vertical plane. Rather, their glenoids are tilted back and angled upward, skyward or more cephalad. This position and orientation aids in their arboreal existence of climbing, swinging and hanging from trees. (figure 35)

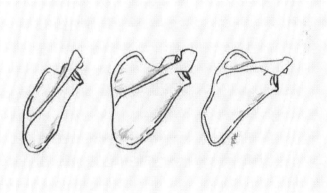

FIGURE 35

As we move towards gorillas and orangutans, their glenoids, while less cephalad (upward) orientated, are slightly more anteverted (rotated forward). Looking at a gorilla skeleton (figure 36), we see that their arms are a bit longer. While gorillas use their hands for dexterity, they still use their upper limbs for ambulation. For this reason, their scapulas are longer and rest on the side of their chest wall. In fact, while they do have clavicles, they are relatively shorter than humans as their shoulders often function in a more protracted-side chest wall position. In fact, all non-humanoid primates have shorter clavicles as compared to humans. In gorillas, in order to match this position of their shoulder, their proximal humerus is more retroverted, meaning twisted backwards. This retroverted orientation allows the humeral head to articulate with the protracted-side chest wall positioned scapula and glenoid while allowing the forearm to function in a frontal plane. Now I know that last point may be a little esoteric, and once again don't waste too much time thinking about it, just realize that we find a more primitive shoulder orientation in our closer relatives.

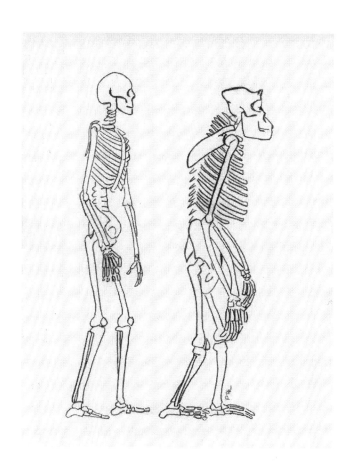

FIGURE 36

Now let us take a look at some of our closer relatives. Anatomic studies and theories examining the shoulders of Homo floresiensis, an early ancestor living 12,000 years ago, and early Homo erectus reveal that they had shorter clavicles and more retroversion torsion to their proximal humeri. These two findings support the fact that their scapulae are more protracted, laterally placed on the chest wall with their glenoids facing anteriorly. This increased humeral torsion allowed their elbows and arms to function in the more advantageous and useful sagital plane rather than a frontal plane. (figure 37)

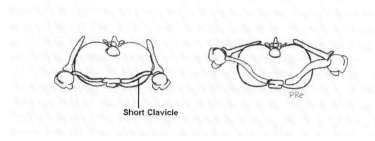

Short Clavicle

FIGURE 37

This orientation is perhaps an intermediate step from the more primitive position to the stance we have as humans with longer clavicles and retracted less retroverted proximal humeri.

So why did we as humans develop this position of scapular retraction, or why was it selected (that is keeping our scapula on the back of our chest walls and the longer clavicles to keep them there)? Well many theories abound: Since we developed our upper limbs to function with more dexterity rather than ambulation, we had to develop more stability with bipedal ambulation and running. That is having longer clavicles and a retracted scapular position allows us to rotate our upper torso and limbs to counteract the motion and torque produced by our legs while running. In addition, this shoulder position allows for better throwing with the arm, a useful factor in hunting and self-defense. Finally, a protracted shoulder dramatically increases the range of motion of our shoulder and usefulness of our arms particularly in a posterior orientation.

Our shoulders developed over many, many years to obtain a position with the scapula retracted on the back of our chest walls, the clavicles to keep them there, and the muscles to stabilize them low against our chest wall posteriorly. In this position, we are least likely to injure ourselves. Initially, we as humans were nomadic hunters and gatherers, and the specialized upper extremity helped us be successful. As we developed larger brains and became more intelligent, we developed a more formal culture and social interaction to pass down the skills and information we learned to the next generation. But among the most influential change that occurred was in the Fertile Crescent over 10,000 years ago with the development of successful agriculture. With the development of productive, reproducible and flourishing agriculture, humans no longer were subjected to being nomadic hunters and settled down in these areas creating towns, cities and a more formalized society. With the larger, more intelligent brains and the highly advanced dexterity in our upper extremities, we were now able to alter our environment to make us more successful and prosperous.

In fact, this allowed us to become less influenced by the environmental forces of evolution and natural selection and instead we adapted the world around us despite some of our own physical limitations. Since that time, we as humans have created an artificial environment in which we live. We have developed such a specialized society in which we work and live, that our bodies, which slowly evolved over millions of years influenced by environmental forces, are not well designed for us to live in this new artificial world we created. We were originally nomadic hunters/gatherers that walked and ran to perform these tasks, sat down to eat and rest, and lay down to sleep. Over an incredibly short period of time, we developed a life style that sits for the large majority of life whether it be working, eating, traveling or socializing. The only true time we walk and run is when we have the need to get somewhere close or have the desire to exercise. We live our lives in front of ourselves, constantly using our anterior chest wall muscles and rarely our back ones. Many of us sit at desks all day, working at a computer. (figure 26) This position leads us to slouch, reach our arms forward and protract our shoulder and in particular our scapulas. Interestingly enough, this is a position that our less evolved ancestors have. Our problem is that the bone structure of our scapulas and humeri as well as their alignment and articulation angle (version) are not appropriate for this position.

We live in this position, constantly at risk for injury because we were not designed to have this alignment. While we may go for years without injury, as our shoulders roll more forward, as our back muscles become weaker, as our posture slouches, we are primed for injury. When we perform an activity overhead or behind us, that our bodies were originally designed to do, we are no longer in the correct alignment. The cascade of injury can begin, and begin the cycle of repetitive injury.

Now it may seem a long way to work through evolution to get to this idea, but it is important to understand this in order to understand injury patterns and prevention.

PAIN and COMMON QUESTIONS

I know that this is an odd title for a section in this book, but it is common reasons why patients present for evaluation and treatment. The pain is so severe that it affects their daily life, activities and sleep and they are concerned and have questions about it. So I have decided to include questions that patients commonly ask and the answers in order to shed some light on these very important issues and questions.

If the problem is my shoulder, then why does it hurt me in my arm? (Pointing to their upper arm, Deltoid area.)

If the problem is my shoulder, then why does it hurt me in my back? (Pointing to the medial edge of their scapula.)

If the problem is my shoulder, then why does it hurt me in my neck? (Pointing to the muscles at the side of their neck.)

These three questions are really related to each other. You experience pain in these areas for a few reasons.

First, a pain in the Deltoid can be referred from the shoulder. This is similar to patients with heart "angina" having pain in their left arm. You have often heard that when a person is having a heart attack, the often feel pain in their left arm. Now clearly their heart is not in their arm but because of cross over nerves that supply the arm and shoulder, people can get a referred pain in the arm, back or neck as a result of problems in the shoulder. In addition, in the lateral part of the arm there is a subacromial bursa which travels for a couple of centimeters underneath the Deltoid. With tendonitis and bursitis, this bursa can get inflamed and irritate the Deltoid above it. With rotator cuff dysfunction, the Deltoid has to do 'extra work' in its compensation for the weakened rotator cuff and this can irritate it.

The pain along the medial border of the scapula and up into the neck are both related to the same cause. When you have a problem with your shoulder, and it drops and rolls forward, the muscles in the back and neck have to do extra work to compensate for the injured cuff muscle. The muscles at particular risk and a site of pain are the Rhomboids and the Levator Scapulae. They are also stretched out because of the scapula's poor posture and position, directly injuring and irritating the muscles. In cases where the shoulder is stiff at the Gleno-humeral joint because of scar or inflammation, the scapula moves more than normal. Since the scapula is moving more, the muscles that move it and stabilize it are being used more and as a result hurt more.

Why are my fingers and hands numb and tingle some times?

Sometimes my whole hand feels numb and I want to shake it out or rub it. Why does that happen?

The first thing a doctor has to do is make sure that the numbness and tingling you feel is not related to a pinched nerve or disc problem in your neck. These usually follow specific anatomic distribution and have more of a burning sensation, electrical shock feeling and weakness. These symptoms are often more constant.

However, shoulder problems can cause patients to have an occasional or intermittent non-specific numbness or funny feeling in their hands that does not present in a specific anatomic distribution. It is usually more vague.

Patients typically say that they want to rub their hands or shake them out. Again this is occasional and not constant. It is often related to shoulder use and often resolves when they pull their shoulder blades/scapulas back and down on their back. The nerves that supply the hand and the arm, start in the neck travel under the collar bone (clavicle), then under the shoulder and down the arm to the hand. When a person has a problem with the shoulder and as a result has some swelling, this swelling can irritate these nerves as they pass under the shoulder. In addition, if you have a shoulder problem, often you roll the shoulder forward, these also tends to pinch the nerves or place them under tension. If you have a stiff shoulder, the abnormal motion your shoulder goes through can cause traction and irritation to these same nerves.

This is a common finding and it is related to the nerves that go to your hand and finger tips. These nerves start at your neck, travel under your clavicle and form a group of nerves called the brachial plexus. From here the plexus separates into distinct nerves that then travel beneath your shoulder and down into the arms, hands and fingers. When your shoulder is injured, a couple of things happen, you drop and roll your shoulder down and forward, and you have inflammation about the joint and muscles themselves. This poor posture places stretch on the brachial plexus and nerves and causes irritation to them. In addition, the swelling about the shoulder further irritates the nerves and causes the strange sensation experienced. The key finding is that it is a non-specific, generalized feeling and doesn't follow a particular anatomic distribution of a single nerve. In those more specific cases, you must make sure that these symptoms are not caused by a pinched nerve in the cervical spine caused by a disc herniation or a more distal nerve compression such as is seen in carpal tunnel syndrome. Careful symptom history taking is essential as well as a careful neurologic exam to rule out these other possible causes for these symptoms.

Why does my elbow hurt so much?

There are many reasons why someone also develops elbow pain. One reason is that when you injure your shoulder, you move the shoulder less and your elbow is overused to compensate. In addition, since you often do not and cannot move your shoulder into the best position to use your elbow, your elbow is now working in a non-normal, non-ideal plane of motion which can lead to injury. When someone has injured their shoulder and it gets stiff, the body compensates by trying to get more rotational motion from the elbow to compensate and as a result, you experience pain.

Why does my shoulder hurt me when I sleep at night?

When you are standing upright, the weight of the arm distracts the shoulder joint downward, taking load off of the irritated cuff tendons and bursa and moving it down and away from the potential of irritation from the acromion and any spur above them. When you lie down, the shoulder pushes up against itself, pinching the cuff bursa and acromion together. When you are awake and upright, and you move, you actively stabilize and splint your arm with the other muscles about your shoulder. When you are asleep, your muscles relax and if you roll or turn in bed, you have no protective conscious muscle splinting and your shoulder moves unopposed leading to further irritation and pain.

One effective way to help with pain at night is to sleep in a more upright position. An upright reading pillow with arm extensions is a great solution. Alternatively, using a couple of pillows as a wedge is another good option. Using a recliner can also be considered.

I hear this popping and crunching in my shoulder when I move it around, does that mean I have a rotator cuff tear?

Possibly, but not usually. Popping and crunching are non-specific findings that are found in any shoulder condition that causes inflammation and or scarring in the bursa. This popping and crunching is caused by the inflamed and or scarred bursa rubbing against itself or other surfaces. In fact, most uninjured shoulders pop or crunch. Put your hand on your un-injured shoulder and move it around. Chances are you will feel or hear popping and crunching. We are more concerned if there is pain that accompanies the crunching or popping.

What should I use? Ice or Heat?

The short answer is to do whatever makes it feel better. The old adage still applies for acute injuries. Use cold packs for 30 minutes every 3-4 hours for the first couple days. Ice the injured muscle or joint for the first 24 to 48 hours, and then use heat to loosen up the muscle.

More specifically, if you are having pain in the shoulder joint, then you ice the shoulder joint. If you are having pain in the muscles around the shoulder, then you should use moist heat on the muscles. Pain in the shoulder is usually a result of swelling or inflammation and ice will help that. Pain in the muscles is usually due to overuse and spasm and moist heat is best to help that.

I say, 'Ice the joint, heat the muscle, but if you tell me the exact opposite works for you, then do that.'

Another helpful hint is to heat and warm up the muscles before a therapy session and then ice the joint after. Most people find that doing their home therapy exercises after a warm shower is beneficial.

Why does a cortisone injection work or help, can I

damage my shoulder by getting one and are they safe (non-intravenous)?

The exact mechanism and pathway by which soft tissue corticosteroid injections work is not perfectly known, other than it decreases inflammation as well as the number of lymphocytes, mast cells and macrophages.

Cortisone injections are safe when they are given in the appropriate settings. Rarely are people allergic to them, more commonly they are allergic to the carrier molecule in the solution. Therefore, a careful history of allergies must be obtained. Some contraindications to cortisone injections include narrow angle glaucoma and uncontrolled diabetes. For other diabetics, they must be informed that their blood sugars can become elevated for a few days and to adjust their medication appropriately. Some people after an injection can feel hyper or flushed in the face for 12-24 hours. This usually subsides quickly but symptoms can be alleviated in most cases with over the counter Tylenol and Benadryl either before or after the injection. When administered appropriately they do not hurt but rarely some patients experience a 'cortisone flare,' when the injected cortisone crystallizes. This is not dangerous but it usually hurts for 2-3days and treated with cold packs and anti-inflammatory medications. Other relative contraindications include a skin discoloration or fat atrophy with previous injections.

The pharmacologic effect of the injection lasts about 4 weeks.

Doesn't cortisone just mask the problem?

A common concern patients have is that cortisone 'masks' the underlying problem, causing them to then over use the shoulder and injure it. They also are concerned it is only a temporary fix.

The goal of the injection is both diagnostic and therapeutic.

When we inject the shoulder with cortisone, we also inject some local numbing medication. If after the injection, the pain goes away, then we know we are definitely in the correct space. However not having initial relief from the injection does not rule out eventual success.

From a therapeutic standpoint, a swollen injured tendon continues to rub on any bone spur that might be present, cannot heal, and does not function appropriately. All of these lead to repeat injury.

The swollen tendon continues to rub on a bone spur. Rubbing on the bone spur causes more irritation and inflammation. More inflammation and swelling of the tendon makes the tendon thicker and then more likely to rub on a bone spur... and the cycle continues. By allowing the cortisone to decrease the swelling and inflammation of the tendon, the tendon gets less thick, and it stops rubbing on the bone spur and the cycle is broken. It is similar in a way to biting the inside of your cheek. Once it swells, you constantly bite it again and again re-injuring and causing more swelling.

The swelling in the tendon chokes off the vascular supply to that tendon. As a result, the cells in the tendon die or become less productive and cannot maintain or repair the injured tendon. As a result, the tendon can degenerate and tear. A swollen inflamed muscle tendon rotator cuff unit can't function and contract appropriately. This leads to micro dynamic instability and further injury.

Can a cortisone injection in my shoulder cause osteoporosis or bone loss?

Prolonged steroid exposure either in oral or intravenous administration can be associated with risk of some bone loss but this has not been seen with appropriately administered occasional musculoskeletal cortisone injections. With musculoskeletal cortisone injections, the injection is really localized to the area injected and very little is absorbed systemically. An occasional cortisone injection into the bursal tissue of the shoulder or Gleno-humeral joint has little risk.

Why doesn't Cortisone work sometimes?

There are many reasons this could be the case. One is that the inflammation and injury are so significant that another injection or dose is needed. Another is that it may not have been administered in the correct location. This is where an ultrasound guided injection may be beneficial in identifying the point of maximal inflammation and delivering the medication to that exact point. It is also possible that the injury is so significant that a procedure is the only thing that will correct it.

In reaction to injury and swelling, our rotator cuff goes through a progression of phases. The first is tendinitis which is inflammation of the tendon. The next is tendinosis, which is the phase when tendon cell death begins making it more difficult to heal. The next is fibrosis where the normal tendon architecture is being replaced with fibrous tissue which is less elastic. During this phase there is little swelling and inflammation. The last can be tendon degeneration and tearing. As you progress through these phases, there is less inflammation in the tendon and an injection is therefore less successful. This is why is it so important to get rid of the swelling in an injured tendon as early and efficiently as possible.

Are there any alternatives to cortisone?

Yes. The most commonly used are cold packs and non-steroidal anti-inflammatory medicines (NSAIDS) such as ibuprofen and naproxen.

Some people have had success with herbal/homeopathic treatments. The one I use most frequently is Arnica. Arnica is derived from a daisy-like mountain flower. It comes in both pill and gel form.

While I know no particular study that proves its success in musculoskeletal treatment, I have many patients who swear by it.

Can acupuncture help my shoulder pain?

Absolutely. In my practice I have seen acupuncture help significantly. I use it mostly to break pain cycles, and muscle spasms. The needling of specific locations and interfere with pain pathways, breaking the reflexive cycles of pain and offer relief. Also the direct needling of an irritated muscle can often break spasm and yield relief.

Some acupuncturists believe that it can reduce inflammation. It is hypothesized that the release of neuropeptides from the nerve endings causes vasodilation, and in addition it is hypothesized that it has anti-inflammatory effects through calcitonine gene-related peptide. It is also suggested that the acupuncture stimulates release and control of other factors such as tumor necrosis factor-alpha and interleukin-10.

While I cannot confirm the benefits with acupuncture directly decreasing inflammation, I do support and use acupuncture to decrease pain cycles and muscle spasm.

Can chiropractors help my shoulder pain?

Absolutely, in my practice I have great relationships with some talented chiropractors. I have found chiropractors that have a good knowledge of the musculo-skeletal system, understand the importance of mechanics and posture and work with their patients in relieving muscle spasms, pain and imbalance can aid in my patients' recovery.

They often have a great understanding of how axial alignment and neck posture can affect shoulder function and pain. But just like finding a good orthopedic surgeon, one must also make sure they find a good chiropractor. Usually the best and most reliable referrals come from your primary care doctor, specialists and friends.

What are trigger points?
Can trigger point injections help relieve the shoulder pain?

Trigger points are hyperirritable points or nodules in skeletal muscles. They are in a way localized micro-muscle spasms. Pain can originate from these point nodules and radiate outwards. Pressing on these trigger points illicit pain and can radiate pain to another location on the body.

Around the shoulder there are three major or most common locations of trigger points. These are:

1-medial to the inferior pole of the scapula

2-medial to the mid body of the scapula

3- between the medial upper end of the scapula and the base of the neck

They can refer pain up the neck or down the arm. They are hypersensitive and cause significant localized pain. The nodule is believed to be an inflammation or 'knot' in the myofascia, or a localized mini center of chronic spasm in the skeletal muscle.

Having an injured shoulder, causes one to protract the shoulder forward and hold it in an awkward position. This abnormal position causes tension and inflammation in the muscles about the scapula and can result in a trigger point.

Initial treatment is focused on a couple of things. First we need to fix the issue with the shoulder, its inflammation and scapular mechanics and posture. This takes tension off the peri-scapular muscles and can help relieve the symptoms. Next work directly on the trigger point. Direct pressure and massage of the trigger point although initially painful, reduces the stress and spasm and can result in significant pain relief. If you don't have a partner to do this for you, you can lean against a wall and place a tennis ball on the trigger point between your scapula and the wall. I often suggest putting a tennis ball in a sock and using that to 'drape' it over your shoulder and places the tennis ball into position. Trigger point self-massage devices are available from many sources online. I have found that application of moist heat to the area also results in relief of pain.

If these initial treatments don't work trigger point injections can be quite helpful. After sterile preparing the skin around the trigger point, a tiny needle is used to inject the nodule with a small amount of local anesthetic medication and occasionally corticosteroid. While similar to acupuncture in needling the spasm and breaking that cycle, the steroid helps to decrease the localized inflammation and help in healing. If a patient does not want to use any steroid, the injection can be done only with the local anesthetic and expect similar results to acupuncture. The local anesthetic paralyzes the micro muscle spasm in the trigger point for a couple of hours and is used to break the cycle of spasm like resetting a fuse.

Why does my shoulder hurt only after I lift my arm up half way and then gets better when my hand is above my head?

This is called the painful arc of motion and it occurs most between 60-120 degrees of elevation. At 60 degrees of elevation, the irritated tendon and bursa are starting their maximum contact with the acromion/spur above it. Once your arm is elevated past 120 degrees, the irritated tendon and bursa have moved away from the acromion and as a result, the pain subsides.

Are there things I should avoid?

This is a complex question. It is usually very activity dependant and where you are in you shoulder health and rehabilitation.

In general terms, you should avoid activities where your hands or arms are held away from your body or repetitive activities above your shoulder. In addition, you should avoid any activity that requires you to place your scapula in an awkward position as it puts you at risk for injury. An example of this is reaching behind you while seated in the driver's seat of the car. I cannot tell you how many people I have treated because they twisted their arm trying to get something off the back seat or the floor behind them in a car. That is a mechanically disadvantageous position.

When returning to weightlifting while recovering from an injury I suggest one focus on exercises below their shoulder with their scapula appropriately seated on their back. Rowing and Lat Pulldowns are excellent rehabilitative exercises as long as the terminal aspect of the exercise is pinching your shoulder blades together. I want patients to avoid bench presses, dips and military presses. These exercises not only produce significant tangential stress across the shoulder articular surface but its end goal of strengthening works to tighten the anterior chest, pulling the scapula forward and up and ultimately into a mechanically disadvantageous position. You will be able to do light exercises on chest press machines if you use the vertical handles, with your hands below your chest. Cables can also be used with low resistance and high repetitions as long as your shoulder blades are set back, and your hands are below your chest. When returning to the gym after recovering, it is probably best to always avoid the use of barbells and instead use dumbbells, machine and cables. Barbells put your shoulder in a bad posture that encourage pinching of the tendons and injury.

What is ultrasound and how is it used in evaluating and treating shoulder injuries?

Are ultrasound guided injections better than standard injections?

Diagnostic Ultrasound uses high frequency sound waves to obtain images of the soft tissue in your body. Most of us have seen it used during pregnancy but it has been getting more use in musculoskeletal imaging over the past decade.

I use it in my practice to evaluate for tears of the rotator cuff, tendonitis, bursitis and other similar conditions. I also use it as a visual inspection of how the tendon may be healing or swelling resolving. It also has the benefit in that it provides real time dynamic imaging of the tendon that we are evaluating. With the patient watching the screen, we can have them move their shoulder and watch the tendon and joint move and see its function and evaluate impingement. The limitations to ultrasound are that in larger arms with dense fat, the images are not as precise and it is harder to evaluate deeper structures. If there is a bone in the way of what we are trying to image, the sound waves bounce off the bone, does not penetrate it and we really cannot get a good evaluation of the structures within the glenohumeral joint. In cases where intra-articular imaging is needed, an MRI is performed which provides an excellent evaluation. In general, get excellent images of the rotator cuff tendons in most cases with diagnostic ultrasound.

Most injections about the shoulder can be done by referencing anatomic landmarks and we have had excellent success with these techniques over many years. However, ultrasound guidance of the injection, when needed, does allow us to precisely localize our injection to the area of maximal inflammation, or to a specific anatomic structure. In addition, it allows us to reliably and accurately perform an injection into the articular space when needed. While most shoulder injections are not significantly uncomfortable, I also find that ultrasound guided injections are much less painful given its ability to observe and confirm proper administration of the medication. Again it is a tool, and when needed has greatly assisted in our treatment. However, many injections can still be, and are, very successful and appropriately given using standard techniques.

What is kinesiology tape?

Kinesiology Tape of Kinesio Tape is a thin, elastic, stretchy tape usually made of cotton with an adhesive backing. It comes in a variety of decorative colors and can come in a simple roll form or preformed cut patterns to better cover a joint or area.

The traditional cloth taping involves circumferentially wrapping an injured joint and has been used to compress, stabilize and support it. The kinesiology tape is used differently.

It is placed in different patterns and tensions across an injured or recovering joint or body area. It is not used as a circumferential wrap, as there is concern that this type of wrapping may limit blood flow necessary for healing as well as limit drainage of swelling. It is used to support the area but also to encourage it to dynamically stay in the desired position as you strengthen the appropriate muscles through rehabilitation. In addition, by placing the dynamic tension across the skin, it provides secondary neuro-feedback to your brain to aid in proprioception (awareness of your body in space). It provides a tactile reminder to you to maintain or obtain the correct posture or mechanical position.

Another benefit of Kinesiology tape is that it can be left on for a few days.

The developer of the tape also believes that the tension the tape places on the skin cells activates a localized endogenous analgesic system. He also believes that the tension produced across the skin and joint creates pressure differentials that aide in draining of lymphatic fluid and swelling.

Scapular posture shirts and braces have been developed to encourage good shoulder posture. The shirts are easy to use and do not require application of tape.

Why do we fix Rotator Cuff Tears?

We fix rotator cuff tears to relieve our patients from pain, allow them to sleep at night, give them full functionality and prevent problems down the line.

We know that there are many people who are walking around, functional for their lifestyle without any pain with an asymptomatic rotator cuff tear that they are completely unaware of. By imaging asymptomatic shoulders with MRI or ultrasound, some studies have shown that roughly 10% of people in their 50's have tears, as do 20% of people in their 60s, 30% in people in their 70s and 50% in people in their 80's. So tearing of the rotator cuff is clearly an attritional degenerative process with age. The question that isn't fully answered is what makes an asymptomatic tear symptomatic.

A study (J Bone Joint Surg Am, 2013 Jul 17;95(14):e101 1-2) followed asymptomatic tears for three years clinically, with ultrasound and MRI. The study found that over 30% converted into symptomatic tears. It was associated with significant increase in tear size and decreased muscle quality. So the progression of the tear led to symptoms.

Most small tears that are stable don't hurt. A tear that is progressing or tearing further does. Imagine that you had a cut on the skin on your arm. If you did not close the laceration, if you stabilized the edges, and the edges did not move or tear, you would not feel any pain. However, if you move the skin around, stressing the skin edges, even slightly tearing, the more it would hurt.

A simplified algorithm I use is based upon the type of tear (degenerative or traumatic), the size of the tear, the health of the patient and their symptoms. In regard to symptoms, patients pretty much present for evaluation if they felt significant pain or felt limited so that pretty much eliminates asymptomatic tears. If someone is very ill or limited functionally, it is unlikely that we would operate on them unless we cannot manage their pain otherwise. Similarly, if they only felt slightly limited in their daily activities and able to sleep well, we usually elect to follow them and support with therapy. If the patient has a small or partial tear that was caused by defined trauma, we try methods of decreasing inflammation and therapy to see if it stabilizes. If it gets worse or fails to improve in 6 months, we usually suggest arthroscopic repair. If a patient has a significant sized tear, which is painful, limits their sleep and functionality, and has had symptoms for a while, we are going to recommend fixing it.

It is clear that tears in the rotator cuff get worse over time. I cannot predict at what rate or over what time period but they will get worse. Like a tear in a flag or sailcloth flapping in the breeze, a rotator cuff tendon with a tear, with use, will get bigger. Larger tears with muscle atrophy are harder to repair, and if they get too big or too atrophied they cannot be fixed. The result can be a chronically painful weak and arthritic shoulder.

If a patient has a significant sized tear, which is

painful, limits their sleep and functionality, and does not resolve with non-operative management, we are going to recommend fixing it. The outcomes of repair are excellent; it fixes the tendon and at least stops the tear progression. Most patients return to full activities. Conversely, the risk of not repairing asymptomatic tears is far too great, often leading to chronic pain, weakness and limited use.

If I have a bone spur in my shoulder, and no symptoms, do I have to have it removed surgically?

No. Between the acromion bone and the coracoid process (another part of the scapula), there exists a ligament called the coraco-acromial ligament. A small percentage of people are 'born with' a hooked shape acromion, but most bone spurs grow with age. The bone spur of the acromion is an aging ossification of this ligament. There is a very simple classification of the acromion's morphology or shape/spur. A Type 1 acromion is flat, without a spur, a Type II acromion has a small to moderate sized curve or spur, and a Type III acromion has a very large hook or spur.

Studies have shown the prevalence of Type I acromion is about 20% and the association with a torn rotator cuff is only 3%. The prevalence of Type II acromion is about 40% and the association with a torn rotator cuff is about 25%. The prevalence of Type III acromion is about 40% and the association with a torn rotator cuff is about 70%. As we age the prevalence of Type II and Type III acromions increase as does the incidence of tears of the rotator cuff.

So what does this tell us? Well as we already know, as we get older, the coraco-acromial ligament progressively ossifies and we are more likely to have a bone spur. Also, as we get older and are more likely to have a bone spur, and we are more likely to have a tear.

But let's look at this from the opposite point of view. There are a significant number of people who have a bone spur and yet have no symptoms, and no torn rotator cuff tendon. Also, there is a small group of patients who have a spur and a torn rotator cuff but have no symptoms what so ever (25-50% of asymptomatic shoulders have a rotator cuff tear, the percentage increases with age).

Non symptomatic patients who have bone spurs do

not have to prophylactically remove them. If you have symptoms of inflammation, tendonitis or bursitis then you might have a bone spur. The bone spur most likely has been there for years prior to you becoming aware you had one and you were without symptoms. If we can decrease your inflammation, fix your motion, mechanics, and strength, and break the cycle of inflammation and injury, you can continue to live your life symptom free and with your bone spur.

However, if your symptoms have gone on for more than 6-9 months, and treatment has not been successful, you should consider a procedure to remove the spur.

Why do we remove acromial bone spurs?
When do you remove an acromial bone spur?

We remove acromial bone spurs when a person has a chronic impingement/bursitis that has not responded to modalities of treatment over an extended period of time. In general, we suggest that a patient try anti-inflammatory methods and Physical Therapy for 6-9 months before considering removing the bone spur.

After about 12 weeks of swelling of the tendon, we

begin to see tendon cell death. We see a progressive avascular thickening of the tendon and fibrosis by 6 months. Eventually this avascular, fibrotic tendon can fail and easily tear.

Simply put, I tell my patients, if your symptoms have been going on for more than 6-9 months, if you have tried at least two cortisone injections, if your shoulder continues to wake you up at night and interfere with your activities of daily living, you are a candidate for arthroscopic spur removal.

If you are having a rotator cuff repair, the bone spur is removed at the same time for a couple of reasons: 1- To remove one of the causes of the tear, 2- To allow room for the healing tendon to move and heal without stress, and 3-The blood from the raw surface of the acromion where the spur was removed, bathes the healing tendon with natural healing growth factors, fibrin and clot, and aids in tendon repair.

Am I too old to have surgery?

At what patient age would you not operate on a shoulder?

When considering having an operation for any reason it is based on many factors. One of these factors is age. But it is not age as a strict limitation, it is health as it is associated with age.

If you are having a problem that limits your quality of life, as long as you are healthy, age as a number, does not influence the decision to have surgery.

What is the difference between Arthroscopy and Laparoscopy?

The word ARTHROSCOPY is derived from arthro-joint and scopy-scope. Basically looking into the joint using a scope. More specifically Arthro comes from the Greek- Arthron and Latin- Artus meaning a joint.

Laparoscopy is derived from laparo- abdomen and scopy-scope. Basically it is looking into the belly or abdomen using a scope. More specifically from the Greek- Laparo meaning flank, soft spot, abdominal wall.

In orthopedics and shoulder surgery we perform arthroscopic procedures while in general surgery they perform laparoscopic procedures.

Besides medicine, what are other ways to control pain after an injury and during recovery?

What does 'relax into the pain' mean?

There are many other ways to help manage pain.

Ice has long been used to help ease pain. The cold constricts the capillaries and limits swelling of the area. In addition, the cold can directly numb the pain fibers and decrease the pain neurotransmitters at the injured area.

Heat is used to decrease muscle spasm and after the initial injury, applied to dilate and open up the capillaries to aide in swelling reduction.

Relaxation methods of deep breathing have been shown in many scenarios to aid in pain relief. Most people are aware of how controlled breathing aides during child birth. In times of pain when it feels like your body is out of control, deep slow breaths allow you to consciously control one physical part of your body. As a result, these simple deep breaths send a message to your brain that you are in control, and you calm down, you start to relax and your stress decreases. As a result, your heart slows down and your blood pressure decreases. Focusing on your breathing also distracts you and your brain from the injured painful area. You can also focus on a part of your body that isn't injured or in pain and move it. Showing your brain that you are in control and have an overall healthy body also helps in relieving pain.

We find that the feeling of helplessness also makes the pain worse. The thought that the pain will never go away compounds the cycle of pain and allows one brain to let your pain get out of your control. The simple knowledge, reinforcement and belief that your pain is temporary and under your control greatly limits its effect upon you.

By relaxing into the pain, you let your shoulders drop back into the correct mechanical postural position and allows your muscles to relax. As a result, the tension in your muscles lessen, spasm settles down, the nerve endings lessen their transmission to your brain and you experience less pain.

Meditation and positive thoughts also aid greatly and have a similar pathway.

How can stress and anxiety make your shoulder pain worse?

Many studies have shown that stress and anxiety directly affects our brain and its neurotransmitters and makes us more sensitive to pain. In direct relation to the shoulder, when a person is anxious or is feeling stressed, they contract their shoulders up and forward and as we know this is a primed position for injury of the shoulder. In addition, a constantly contracted muscle in a steady state of spasm cannot contract and move appropriately. Also, this contracted shoulder state, makes it more likely to stiffen up and scarring can set in the capsule.

We can relive spasm and anxiety with the following methods:

-Apply moist heat to the muscles.

-Moving and being active also distracts your brain and helps to decrease stress levels.

-Getting more sleep at night allows you to be better able to cope with stress.

-The use of meditation, deep breathing exercises, and thought distraction are well proven methods to decrease both stress and anxiety.

-Also, you should always seek support, talk to your partner or friend and if needed your physician about the factors in life which are stress and anxiety producers. In some cases, patients may need to be prescribed short term antidepressants or anxiolytics. The short term use of these medications can be used to get us over the hump of anxiety associated with injury or surgery and aide in a quicker recovery. This can be a good starting point to discuss our anxiety and stress with our primary care physician.

What does 'decrease the inflammatory load' mean?

Inflammation in the shoulder can cause significant pain. Resolving the inflammation, resolves the pain. Sometimes people with arthritis have significant swelling and they are not a candidate for shoulder replacement due to age, choice or other factors. If we can decrease the stresses that the shoulder experiences and partially decrease the inflammation, we might be able to decrease the pain they experience to a tolerable level. This can be done by increasing the shoulder flexibility, breaking the cycle of inflammation with cortisone injections or NSAIDs, strengthening the shoulder muscles, and sometimes surgically cleaning up loose pieces and bone spurs with an arthroscopic procedure. While these methods do not eliminate the arthritis, by 'decreasing the inflammatory load,' we can lower their pain levels, sometimes significantly to a manageable level.

What is an NSAID?
Are Tylenol(acetaminophen) , Advil (ibuprofen) and Aleve (naproxen) the same?

Acetaminophen decreases pain and fever, while NSAIDs decrease swelling, pain and has a varying effect on reducing fever depending on which one you take.

Acetaminophen(Tylenol) primarily works in our brains by blocking the messages returning from our body that produce pain. In addition, it has an effect on parts of the brain that influences and helps to reduce fever.

Ibuprofen (Advil, Motrin), Naproxen Sodium(Aleve), Celecoxib(Celebrex) and Aspirin all belong to a class of medications called NSAIDs (Non-Steroidal Anti-Inflammatory Drugs). These medications work in our body by influencing the production of chemicals called prostaglandins. The particular prostaglandins targeted by the NSAIDs are called Cox-1 and Cox-2 enzymes. These prostaglandins cause inflammation and also amplify the nerve signals back to our brain that results in the feeling of pain. By blocking the production of these prostaglandins, NSAIDs can reduce swelling and pain. While Ibuprofen and Naproxen Sodium inhibit the production of both Cox-1 and Cox-2, Aspirin inhibits Cox-1 much more than Cox-2 and Celecoxib selectively inhibits Cox-2. Cox-2 is primarily responsible for inflammation and pain while Cox-1 induces clot formation thereby influencing bleeding and it also induces the production of a protective mucus in our stomachs and limits pepsin production. Prostaglandin E2 is responsible for inducing a fever response in our body. A particular NSAID's effect on E2 production, helps to reduce fever in our body.

Major side effects of Acetaminophen are that at high doses it can be toxic to our liver. Depending on which NSAID you take, they can cause stomach ulcers, stomach pain, thinning of the blood and certain NSAIDs can actually increase your risk of cardiac events.

Why does it take so long to recovery from a shoulder injury?

Why does it take so long to recover from a shoulder Rotator Cuff repair?

In general terms many things have to happen. In the case of a tendonitis or bursitis the following events need to happen. First, the swelling in the tendon and bursa need to resolve. Second, once that swelling resolves, the cells in the tendon (fibroblasts/tenocytes) need to recover. With the swelling resolved the nutrients can feed the cells again and they can perform their reparative process. Next, with the tendons healing, the rotator cuff muscles will start firing and functioning appropriately and contract in the appropriate order. As you know, not only do your muscles have to contract and work, in the shoulder, they have to contract in appropriate sequence. Lastly, these muscles need to regain their strength. And on top of all that, your shoulder needs to regain its full flexibility back to allow it to move smoothly and through full function.

In the best case scenario, it will take at least 3-4 months to recover from a bursitis or tendonitis and sometimes longer.

When the rotator cuff is torn and repaired the same factors have to occur but on a bigger level. In simple terms, I tell my patients that it takes 10-12 weeks for the repaired tendon to heal and then another 10-12 weeks for your strength to recover. The longer the period of time you were living with a torn tendon, the longer it takes for the muscle to strengthen. Think about it, if the tendon isn't attached to the humerus of the shoulder, it is usually not firing correctly and sometimes, if the tear is large, it doesn't contract at all. It isn't being stretched and it gets stiff and scarred in. It can take up to a year to regain full range of motion especially in rotation, and in particular reaching your arm behind your back.

Considering strength, flexibility, posture and mechanics, which is the most important to your shoulder health and recovery?

Why are my doctor and therapist spending so much time on posture and stretching and little if any time on strengthening of my shoulder?

I tell my patients that in order of importance you

need to focus on posture, then flexibility, then mechanics and lastly strength.

Unless you obtain correct posture, you will continue to injure yourself. Until you obtain good flexibility you cannot perform the tasks to get good mechanics. Lastly, if you strengthen before you have the first three, then you overload your shoulder with improper mechanics, lack of flexibility and poor posture. Then, you will never get better and just reinforce the injury cycle instead. While we immediately start on scapular retraction and positioning strengthening, we do not introduce shoulder rotator cuff and secondary stabilizer strengthening until 6-8 weeks after the surgery and only if the first three goals have been successfully met.

When I stretch, it hurts. At what point should I stop?

In order to get better, do I need to push through the pain?

When it comes to stretching, the general rule is slow gentle persistence. Meaning that you move slowly through the motion, there is no aggressive forcing, and when you get to the limit, you push a little more and then hold it for a few seconds. Also, it is okay to work with a dull ache, but not a sharp stabbing pain.

If you feel a sharp pain, you should stop and reposition. Stretching that causes significant pain only causes your shoulder to become more reactive, swollen and stiffer. Stretching that causes you to have significant pain the next day, probably is actually irritating the area.

A good method I teach is that when you get to the point of pain, hold it for a few seconds, take two deep slow breaths, and then relax and see if you can release into the position and where you want to get to. As a trick, when you feel that you are not progressing, try to think of it differently. Think of it not as a forceful stretching, rather a relaxation and releasing of stresses.

In general, you can work and stretch with a dull ache; you stop with sharp stabbing pain.

I hear a popping in my shoulder, is that bad?

All joints pop and crack to some degree. Often we are not aware of it until we injure that joint and pay more attention to it. So popping and cracking doesn't mean anything in and of itself. However, a pop, a crunch or a clunk that results in pain does need to be addressed and is usually a sign of swelling, poor mechanics or other issues that should be discussed with your doctor or therapist.

When should I do my exercises?

Whenever you can. I understand, we all lead lives that are way too busy, and life gets in the way of us taking care of ourselves. Just try and find some time that works for you. If you are looking for some particular guidance, the best thing for us to do is work out every day of the week in some manner. Find a complete routine of all exercises you want to do, and then spread them out throughout the week. You can do the same stretch everyday but you should not repeat the same strengthening exercise in consecutive days.

For those of us who cannot arrange a full week exercise schedule, I recommend exercising four days a week. When patients ask me how to remember and stay on top of it, I recommend that they exercise on the two groups of days of the week that start with the same letter:

T-T, S-S: Tuesday, Thursday, Saturday, Sunday.

How does my lower extremities/hips and knees effect my shoulder?

Why do my doctor and therapist have me stretch my hips and knees?

Tightness and lack of flexibility in your legs throws your alignment out of position and causes you to roll your shoulders forward. This protracted position primes your shoulder for injury as it places your shoulder in a mechanical disadvantage. This position rolls your scapula forward and tilts the acromion (and any spur) into your rotator cuff.

You can understand this by standing up and looking at your posture in a mirror and turning sideways to view your body's profile. Bend your knees and watch what happens. When you bend your knees, your pelvis rolls backward, your back hunches over, your shoulders roll forward on your back and head tilts forward. This happens because in the side view, or sagittal plane, your head needs to line up over your shoulders, pelvis, knees and feet. In this position, your center of mass and axial alignment is appropriate. When you bend your knees forward, it shifts your center alignment/weight forward, your pelvis pushes back to counter balance that, and as a result your back hunches over and rolls your shoulders forward to bring that center alignment and weight balance over your feet. If you have tight hamstrings and tight anterior hip flexors, your body tends to assume this position and as a result makes it harder to maintain your shoulders retracted back and down on your chest wall. This makes it harder to recover from an injury.

With that in mind, expand that thought to your seated work position. The more you slouch, the more your shoulders roll forward and that prolonged seated positioning encourages tight hamstrings and hip flexors and as a result poor posture when you stand.

With that knowledge you can see how keeping your knees and hips flexible can indirectly effect and improve your scapular posture and thereby shoulder position.

Is there a simple way I can remember or remind myself of correct shoulder and scapular position?

Your shoulders should be roughly in line with your

ears. While sitting, standing and walking, your shoulder blades should sit back and down not under tension but relaxed on your back. I have three things that I do and teach my patients to do throughout the day.

1-A couple times a day, pretend that you are cracking a dozen eggs between your shoulder blades, and then dropping them on the ground behind you. You do this by pinching and holding your shoulder blades together, then move them downward and release the pinch. This breaks any spasm and mentally reinforces correct position.

2-While you are walking around; imagine that you are gently holding a large grape fruit or melon between your shoulder blades. Again not under tension just gently. This helps us develop muscle memory.

3-When we are still confused about correct position, I suggest using farmer's thumbs. Standing with your arms at your side, bend your elbows and put your thumbs under your armpits. This is similar to pretending to flap your arms like a chicken. With your thumbs still in your armpits, bring your elbows back down to your side. Keeping your shoulder blades back, release your thumbs to your side. This will almost uniformly place your shoulder blades in correct position.

What is the best and worst position to sleep in?

All sleeping positions have their pros and cons. While sleeping on your back makes snoring and sleep apnea more likely, sleeping on one's stomach places pressure on your belly and can affect breathing.

With regard to shoulder health, the worst position you can sleep in is with your hand and arm above your head regardless if it is on your back, belly, or side.

While recovering from shoulder injury the best position to sleep in is slightly upright with your injured arm resting on your lap with neutral scapular shoulder retraction. This can be accomplished using a couple of pillows, a reading wedge or recliner and a small pillow supporting your elbow and upper arm. This position unloads your shoulder and is usually the most comfortable.

When asked if it is 'okay' to sleep on your injured shoulder, or should you sleep on the non-injured shoulder, I recommend you do whatever is most comfortable. Most shoulder pain is worse when you lie down, and it often doesn't matter which side you sleep on.

How can I remember what exercises are good or bad for my shoulder?

If an exercise's primary goal is to pull your shoulders and scapulas back and down, or strengthen your back, then they are generally good. If the primary goal is to tighten your anterior chest, or pull your shoulders forward, then they are generally bad or place your shoulder at risk.

Some simple examples of good exercises are lat pull downs, rows and scapular pinches, and reverse flys. Some examples of exercises that potentially can place your shoulder at risk are bench presses, military presses and dips.

If you first set your shoulder blades back and down on your back chest wall, and then perform the exercise, it should be it generally safe.

INJURY PREVENTION
MAINTAINING A GOOD SHOULDER HEALTH

In this section I introduce an exercise program that will retrain and then maintain your shoulder in good flexibility, muscle strength and balance, and posture. The program will include flexibility and postural exercises to help your body obtain and maintain the correct posture and mechanics to prevent and help cure injuries. These exercises will also include exercises for your back and lower extremities as they also play a role in your posture which indirectly affect your shoulder.

The Primary Flow Pathway has a simple goal. Its purpose is to provide you simple stretching, isometric and postural exercises that you can do anywhere, on a regular basis that helps you obtain and maintain shoulder flexibility, postural positioning and mechanics, and good shoulder health. The primary pathway alone is sufficient for most people in obtaining our goal of a healthy shoulder.

The secondary pathway is a more traditional program of specific stretches, isometrics and strengthening exercises. This program will add a focus on dynamic strengthening of the muscles that provide secondary dynamic stabilization of our shoulder, in particular the gleno-humeral joint.

Last in the series of exercises is the Basic Five. These are the simplest basic five exercises that can be done anywhere. These are the simplest of stretching and postural exercises to help obtain and maintain good shoulder health even in the injured shoulder. I would rather you do five basic exercises regularly than to never do a comprehensive program.

The key to any program is doing them. Once it gets too involved, oppressive or time consuming, we are less likely to perform them. It is better to do five exercises regularly then a comprehensive 20 exercise program almost never. Choose the phase and level that causes no pain and that you feel comfortable doing. It is perfectly appropriate to alternate programs during the week or whenever you want.

Before introducing the programs, I will explain types of stretching and muscle exercise. I also include a work station review and education. This consists of an education portion of correct posture and ergonomics of work station set up to help prevent injuries.

A recurrent theme that you will repeatedly notice is the term: 'obtain and maintain.' That is purposefully done as a key to recovering from injury and preventing injuries is the ability to obtain and maintain correct shoulder posture, mechanics and motion.

When we consider shoulder health, I list the importance of different factors in recovery from injury as well as the prevention of injury. Patients always focus on their strength as the key to their success, as it seems to be an obvious solution, in that, 'if I am injured I need to increase my strength.' It is also an observable measure that most people can follow. They are often surprised when I tell them that strength, by itself, is the least important of all aspects of shoulder health and recovery. I list the priority of focus as: Posture, flexibility, mechanics and strength last. Now these independent focuses are arguably interconnected, but the point is made, if you have bad posture and mechanics, it doesn't matter how strong you are. In fact, your increased strength can lead to more injury. If you have good posture, flexibility and mechanics you are less like to injure yourself and more likely to recover as long as you have adequate strength.

While good posture and mechanics do depend on strength, more often it depends more on flexibility and the ability to obtain, and then maintain correct posture and mechanics.

STRETCHING

Stretching is an important component of any muscle or joint in the body but in particular in regard to the shoulder. First, a flexible joint capsule decreases the joint reactive forces our articular cartilage experiences at rest and with motion. This decreases pain as well as decreases the risk of and helps to potentially slow the progression of arthritis. Second, a flexible joint moves smoothly and appropriately. A stiff joint causes our humeral head to rotate and coil upwards with arm motion. This causes our rotator cuff to hit the acromion above it. (Please refer back to the section on Adhesive Capsulitis/Frozen Shoulder for a more detailed explanation)

In regard to muscle flexibility, a tightened shortened

muscle cannot work efficiently. Conversely, an over tensioned muscle or tendon is also at risk for easy overload and tearing, therefore muscle and tendon flexibility is very important.

Good examples in our shoulders are our pectoralis muscles which start on our anterior chest wall, travel outwards and insert onto our upper arm. When this muscle group is particularly tight, it drags our shoulders and scapulas (shoulder blades) to that unhealthy elevated and protracted state that we have talked about. It rolls our shoulders forward into that risk potential unhealthy posture. The result is all the problems that we know that are associated with that position.

In regard to other muscles in the body, tight muscles and tendons in areas that seem remote and far away from the shoulder can have a deleterious effect. In particular the hip flexors, quadriceps, hamstrings and gastrocnemious (Achilles Tendon) play a significant role in axial alignment, posture and resultant shoulder position and posture.

Looking at the body from the side, the correct axial alignment is our head, chest and pelvis aligned over our feet. In this position our shoulder blades sit appropriately retracted and depressed on our upper back. When our Hamstrings and Gastrocnenious/Achilles are tight, our knees bend slightly in its rested state. When our quadriceps and hip flexors are tight, it causes our hips to also want to flex. The result of both of these is that it throws our axial alignment posterior of correct and resultantly, our upper back hunches forward and our shoulders, and scapulas roll up and forward (protract). (figure 25) This sets us up for shoulder injuries. This fact reinforces the importance of flexibility of these seemingly remote muscles and tendon and why if you are working on flexibility to prevent shoulder injuries, one needs to include your lower extremities as well as your shoulders.

In addition, if we are working on strengthening to prevent shoulder injuries, we also must include strengthening of our core musculature and lower extremity strength for similar reasons.

STRENGTHENING

We strengthen the injured muscle to recover the

atrophy and dysfunction from injury. We strengthen the muscles around the injured, or weakened one to protect it while it heals. The muscles that co-contract, and share a functional movement with the injured ones are the ones we focus on to strengthen. This is so they can compensate for and protect the injured muscle while it heals. Other times, we strengthen our muscles to help obtain and maintain the correct posture and mechanics to aid in healing. But, what I find equally as important, is that we strengthen our muscle groups to maintain appropriate mechanics and posture to prevent injury.

In regard to the shoulder, we need to focus on the muscles that bring our scapulas back and down. In general, any exercise that retracts our shoulder blades and keeps them posterior are good, any exercise that brings them forward and protracted are for the most part unnecessary. A good example of an exercise to bring your shoulder blades back are seated rows. An example of an exercise that brings our shoulders forward is a bench press.

For most people, most everything they do in daily life already uses anterior chest wall muscles and very few life activities work the muscles that hold our shoulders back in correct position. I often say to my patients that we live our lives in front of us and rarely take care of what is behind us.

The anterior chest muscles are bigger, stronger and strengthen quicker than our back, scapular retracting muscles, therefore any exercise to strengthen them worsens our posture. For patients who insist on doing bench presses, I encourage them to use lighter weights, and for every one repetition of anterior strengthening they do, they should do 2 posterior scapular stabilizing or retracting exercises.

As a full complement to a balanced program, a program should also include addressing our body's lower extremities and core musculature. The goal is to increase our strength and endurance in setting up our entire body to obtain and maintain the correct axial alignment which in turn helps our shoulders obtain and maintain theirs more easily.

Core strengthening is an important aspect of any program to obtain or maintain healthy posture and mechanics. When we refer to 'core strengthening,' we focus on the muscles that stabilize our axial spine and keep it in appropriate alignment and endurance condition. As the scapula is the platform from which the shoulder functions from, the axial spine is the central platform from which the scapula functions from. To that end, a core strengthening program should be an advanced part of any program to recover from injury or prevent one.

TYPES OF MUSCLE STRENGTHENING

ISOMETRIC

An isometric exercise is an exercise in which no movement occurs. An example is holding a weight in a semi-contracted and motionless state for a period of time. An isometric exercise is typically performed as an anaerobic exercise (does not need increased oxygen production) because it is done only for a few seconds and it involves static contraction of muscles. In this exercise, the muscle length remains the same. Iso (same/one) metric (length). An example is pushing against the wall. One of the biggest benefits of isometric exercise is that one can do it without the aid of any equipment and they are simple. It is basically pushing or trying to move an immovable object.

Isometrics are pure "muscle" contractions that place the stress entirely on the muscle fibers not the joints. One can recruit nearly all the muscle fibers during a maximal isometric contraction - something that doesn't happen with regular eccentric and concentric exercise. The more muscles you recruit and stress/strain, the more healing and muscle growth can as a result occur. The force the muscles see is immediate and not dispersed over a range of motion. They are efficient and muscle specific, meaning that you can more effectively isolate the muscle you want to strengthen.

Since the joint that the muscle controls is not being moved, the tendon associated with that muscle is not being stressed nor is the joint. For that reason, isometric exercises are particularly beneficial in exercising around injured tendons and joints.

DYNAMIC BAND AND TUBES

Dynamic bands are an exercise routine that uses resistive bands or tubes. It strengthens the muscle through a range of motion, but also relies on the co-contraction of other muscles acting across that joint to balance the forces. That is in addition to working the muscle you are interested in, it also exercises and improves the function in the cooperation of opposing and assisting muscle groups. They help on balancing the joint muscle reactive forces and can help with core strengthening. It is a dynamic, balanced and fluid exercise program.

Perhaps the biggest benefit of theraband resistive tubing exercises is that they are versatile, lightweight, portable and inexpensive. They can be done at work or during travel or in the bedroom while one watches TV. Like isometrics, they are simple.

LIGHT WEIGHTS

Most people when they think of weights, focus on how much weight they can push, pull or use. It is ego boosting and also an objective measure of progress. However, the goal of high weight often leads to poor form, imbalance and injury.

People should focus on form function, mechanics and posture and limit the amount of weight. A biceps curl performed with the appropriate scapular posture, axial alignment and controlled contraction is more beneficial and therapeutic when performed with 5 pounds than a 20-pound curl with none of the above.

The use of light weights and more repetitions, increases resting tone, increases endurance and is a more efficient use of aerobic energy. Heavy weight lifting is better for short bursts of contraction and anaerobic muscle contraction.

For that reason and others, people should focus on the use of light weights and more repetitions. Light weights also are preferable as they are less expensive than, and more portable than heavy weights.

WORK STATION EVALUATION

Our work stations (desks, computer stations, work areas, etc...) are quite dangerous places. Dangerous because the position that we sit in as we work, sets us up for injury. This poor position usually starts with how we sit and what we sit in. In addition, the way computer screens, keys pads and mouse are positioned and arranged, are usually not ergonomic. These factors encourage us to hunch our backs, and shrug and roll our shoulders up and forward. This is the exact opposite position which we want them to be maintained.

You want to sit in a position where your hips and knees are bent comfortably at 90 degrees each. You want to sit upright with your lower back, the lumbar area, supported recreating the correct axial alignment of 'lumbar lordosis.' Recreating and supporting this normal lumbar lordosis, as a result, automatically encourages your shoulder blades to roll backward and down on your upper back. Flexing your hips and knees to 90 degrees also encourages the correct lumbar lordosis as it relaxes the tension on your hip muscles which takes tension off your pelvis and low back.

You want the top of your computer screen to be at eye level so your eyes rest at the horizontal mid point of the screen or the midpoint of whichever part of the screen you view the most. This is more difficult if you use a laptop on a desk.

The optimal position of the desk height is a little controversial. From an ergonomic position, the desk height should be the height at which your hands rest parallel to the floor with your upper arms by your side and elbows bent to 90 degrees. However, this is a little low for most people's optimal visual focal length, so often people will have their desk height a couple of inches higher than described above. What is important is that your computer keyboard be placed at the appropriate level as described above. The keyboard should be placed at a level that you are not reaching more than 10 to 15 degrees forward to utilize it. In order to achieve this position, people either raise their chair height or more commonly, use a keyboard tray that is attached under your desk top.

The next common source of shoulder injury is the computer mouse. For such a harmless appearing object its use can cause a great deal of shoulder problems. The first reason is that most people's desk height is too high. Next, they often have their mouse pad deep onto the desk top and since most people are right handed, their paper work dominates the center right of the desk field and the mouse pad is often placed to the right of this. This causes most people to have to reach forward and to the right to use their mouse. In this position, your shoulder blade rolls forward, tilting your acromion down onto your rotator cuff and grinds it into the rotator cuff as you move your mouse around. To correct this, you have a couple of options. You can correct your desk height and move your mouse pad closer to your body and more centrally located on the desk top. If this is not optimal for your work space, you can also get an under desk mounted attachment that can bring it next to your keypad.

What I often recommend is getting rid of your mouse all together and switching to a track ball or track pad instead and place it in the position described above. The track ball and track pad have the benefit that you don't have to move your arm and shoulder around to move the cursor and thereby you avoid rubbing your rotator cuff on the undersurface of the acromion.

The last thing you need to address are your feet. With everything else set and your knees and hips bent to 90 degrees, you want to support your feet to encourage this alignment. If needed, a foot rest can be used if your legs are short or if your legs are long, simply straightening your knees to 70 degrees will suffice.

This position aids in preventing shoulder injuries and also helps to prevent neck and upper and lower back strains.

I encourage my patients to do the Basic Five Exercises in their office. Of course most are not able to do the child's pose at work, but the others are perfectly appropriate in most situations. In fact, I encourage my patients to do the scapular squeezing exercises as they walk around the office.

PRIMARY FLOW PATHWAY

The primary flow pathway is a variant of yoga. It involves a step by step process that transitions from one exercise to another. They are grouped into sections of similar exercises or poses. They are meant to be done together as a program. However, you can choose to do the sections that you like the best or get the most out of.

Begin Primary Flow Pathway:

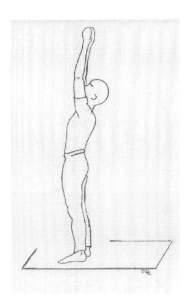

1-Stand with arms by side. This is your starting position. Inhale and while you exhale, bring your shoulder blades back and down on your back.

2-Inhale and while you breath in, raise your hands from your sides over your head and reach as high and as far back as you can. Remember to keep your shoulder blades down, away from your ears. Hold your breath in this position for a count of three.

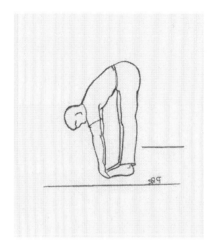

3-Exhale and while you are exhaling, bring your hands downwards, with your elbows fully extended, bend at your hips and touch your toes. Hold this exhaled breath and position for a count of three,

4-Now inhale and stand upright and return to your starting position.

Repeat this cycle 3 times.

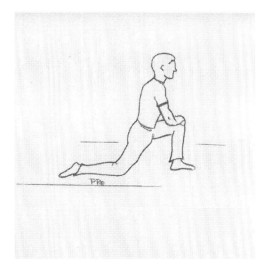

1-Stand with arms by side. This is your starting position. Inhale and while you exhale, bring your shoulder blades back and down on your back and place your hands on your hips.

2-Inhale deeply and while you then exhale, step your right leg forward into a lunge position keeping your right knee and ankle bent at 90 degrees, your shoulder blades pinched back and your left knee straight. Hold this exhaled breath and position for a count of three.

3-Inhale, bring your left leg forward next to your right and return to starting position. Exhale and turn around.

4- Inhale and while you exhale, bring your shoulder blades back and down on your back and place your hands on your hips.

5- Inhale deeply and while you then exhale, step your left leg forward into a lunge position keeping your left knee and ankle bent at 90 degrees, your shoulder blades pinched back and your right knee straight. Hold this exhaled breath and position for a count of three.

6-Inhale, bring your right leg forward next to your left and return to starting position. Exhale and turn around.

Repeat this cycle 3 times.

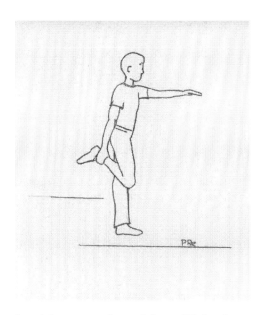

1-Stand with arms by side. This is your starting position. Inhale and while you exhale, bring your shoulder blades back and down on your back.

2-Inhale, and while you inhale, bend your left knee, bring your left heel to your buttocks and grab the top of your foot or your ankle with your left hand. Exhale. For added difficulty, as you exhale, extend your right arm forward and reach outward as you lift with your left hand pulling your left foot and leg higher. Hold this exhaled breath and position for a count of three.

3-Inhale and return to starting position. Exhale and while you exhale, pinch your shoulder blades together and lower them down on your back.

4- Inhale, and while you inhale, bend your right knee, bring your right heel to your buttocks and grab the top of your foot or ankle with your right hand. Exhale. For added difficulty, as you exhale, extend your left arm forward and reach outward as you lift with your right hand pulling your right foot and leg higher. Hold this exhaled breath and position for a count of three.

5- Inhale and return to starting position. Exhale and while you exhale, pinch your shoulder blades together and lower them down on your back.

Repeat this cycle 3 times.

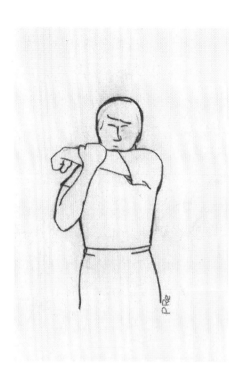

1-Stand with arms by side. This is your starting position. Inhale and while you exhale, bring your shoulder blades back and down on your back.

2-Inhale, and while you are inhaling, bring your right arm across your upper body, under your chin and reach to your left, with your left hand, grab your right elbow and gently pull as you exhale. Hold this exhaled breath and position for a count of five.

3-Inhale and switch sides. While you are inhaling, bring your left arm across your upper body, under your chin and reach to your right. With your right hand, grab your left elbow and gently pull as you exhale. Hold this exhaled breath and position for a count of five.

Repeat this cycle 3 times.

4- Inhale and return to starting position. Exhale and while you exhale, pinch your shoulder blades together and lower them down on your back.

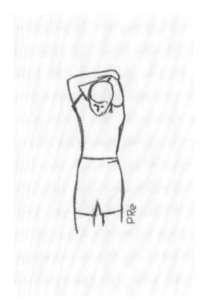

1-Stand with arms by side. This is your starting position. Inhale and while you exhale, bring your shoulder blades back and down on your back.

2-Inhale, and while you are inhaling, reach your right hand and arm overhead, fully extend straight up. Bend your right elbow, bringing your right hand behind your head. Bring your left arm over head and with your left hand grab your right elbow. Exhale while pulling with your left arm down, bringing your right between your shoulder blades. Hold this exhaled breath and position for a count of five.

3-Inhale and switch sides. While you are inhaling, reach your left hand and arm overhead, fully extend straight up. Bend your left elbow, bringing your left hand behind your head. Bring your right arm over head and with your right hand grab your left elbow. Exhale while pulling with your right arm down, bringing your left between your shoulder blades. Hold this exhaled breath and position for a count of five.

Repeat this cycle 3 times.

4- Inhale and return to starting position. Exhale and while you exhale, pinch your shoulder blades together and lower them down on your back.

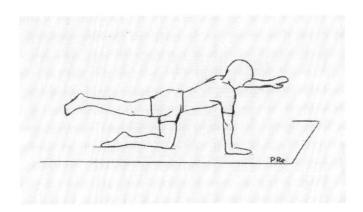

1-Stand with arms by side. This is your starting position. Inhale and while you exhale, bring your shoulder blades back and down on your back.

2-Inhale. While you exhale bring your right foot back, while you kneel on your right knee, bring both hands down to the ground and then bring your left foot back and kneel on your left knee. You are now on all fours.

3-Inhale. While you inhale, bring your right arm up and reach in front of you and extend your left leg back to reach behind you at the same time. Try to reach as far forward as you can with your right hand, and reach as far backwards with your left foot. Hold this position and breath for a count of 5. Exhale and return to your all four position.

4-Inhale. While you inhale, bring your left arm up

and reach in front of you and extend your right leg back to reach behind you at the same time. Try to reach as far forward as you can with your left hand, and reach as far backwards with your right foot. Hold this position and breath for a count of 5. Exhale and return to your all four position.

Repeat this cycle (#3 and 4) 3 times.

1-Staying in your kneeling all four position, inhale and when you exhale pull your shoulder blades back and down.

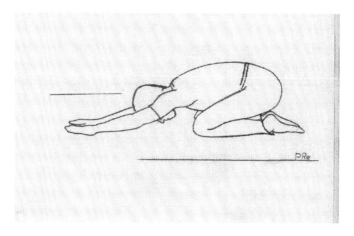

2-Inhale, and when you exhale slowly slide your weight backwards to sit on your heels and extend your hands forward. This is classic child's pose. Try to sit deeper while extending your hands as far forward on the ground as they can go. Hold this position and exhaled breath for a count of 5.

3-Inhale and return to your kneeling all four position, when you exhale pull your shoulder blades back and down.

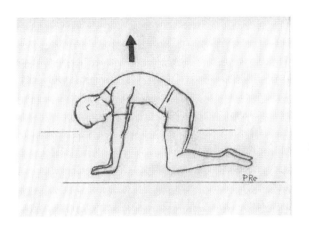

4-Inhale, and while you inhale, hunch your back as much as possible. Hold this position and inhaled breath for a count of 5. Exhale, flatten your back and return to your resting all four kneeling position. Repeat this 3 times

5-Inhale, and when you exhale slowly slide your weight backwards to sit on your heels and extend your hands forward. This is classic child's pose. Try to sit deeper while extending your hands as far forward on the ground as they can go. Hold this position and exhaled breath for a count of 5.

6- Inhale and return to your kneeling all four position, when you exhale pull your shoulder blades back and down.

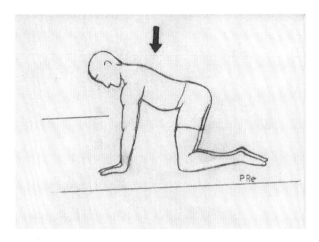

7-Inhale. Lock your wrists elbows and shoulders. While you exhale, drop your chest forward, allowing your shoulder blades to push further backwards. Hold this breath and position for a count of three. Repeat this 3 times.

8-Inhale, and when you exhale slowly slide your weight backwards to sit on your heels and extend your hands forward. This is classic child's pose. Try to sit deeper while extending your hands as far forward on the ground as they can go. Hold this position and exhaled breath for a count of 5.

9-Inhale and return to your kneeling all four

position, when you exhale pull your shoulder blades back and down.

1-Inhale and stand up placing your arms by your side. This is your starting position. Exhale and while you exhale, bring your shoulder blades back and down on your back.

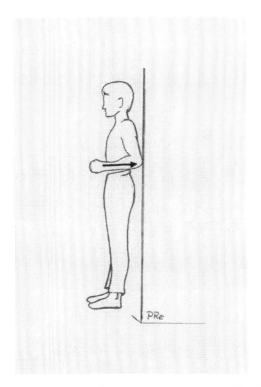

2-Stand with your back against a wall. Bend your elbows 90 degrees and place your elbows against the wall behind you. Inhale while you push your elbows back, pinch your shoulder blades together, lifting your body away from the wall. Hold your breath and this position for a count of three. While you exhale relax your arms returning your back to the wall. This is a back wall push up. Do three sets of ten.

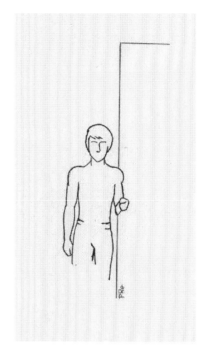

3-Turn to your right placing your 90-degree bent elbow and arm against the wall. While you inhale, rotate your right forearm against the wall exerting constant pressure. Hold your breath and this position for a count of three. Exhale and relax. Do three sets of ten.

4-Turn to your left, placing your 90-degree bent elbow and arm against the wall. While you inhale, rotate your left forearm against the wall exerting constant pressure. Hold your breath and this position for a count of three. Exhale and relax. Do three sets of ten.

5-Inhale and return to your starting position with your arms by your side. Inhale and while you exhale, bring your shoulder blades back and down on your back.

6-Bend your elbows and arms in front of you. Make a fist with your right hand and place it into your left palm. Inhale and push them together. Hold your breath and position for a count of 2. Relax and exhale leaving your hands touching. Do two sets of ten.

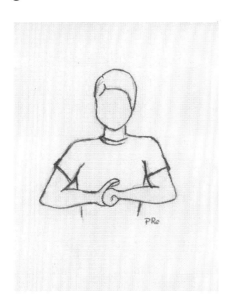

7-Now make a fist with your left hand and place it into your right palm. Inhale and push them together. Hold your breath and position for a count of 2. Relax and exhale leaving your hands touching. Do two sets of ten.

8-Inhale and return to your starting position with your arms by your side. Inhale and while you exhale, bring your shoulder blades back and down on your back.

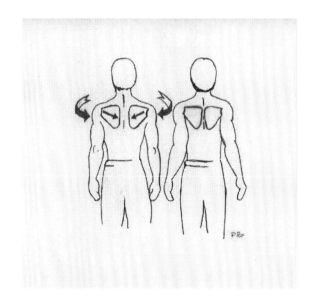

9-Keep your arms by your side. While you inhale, pinch your shoulder blades together as if you were cracking an egg between your shoulder blades. Hold for a count of 2, exhale and relax. Do three sets of ten.

10-Inhale and return to your starting position with your arms by your side. Inhale and while you exhale, bring your shoulder blades back and down on your back.

11-Inhale, and while you exhale, sit down and then lay flat on your back.

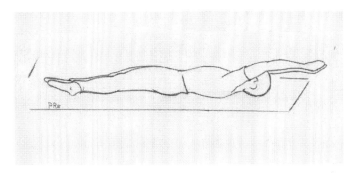

12-Inhale and raise both hands over your head and stretch out along the floor as much as you can. Reaching further away from your head with your hands and away from your body with your toes, hold your breath and this position for a count of ten. Exhale, and relax bringing your hands back down and to your side.

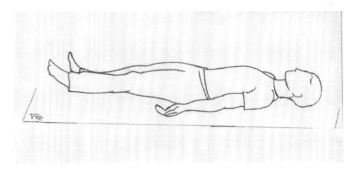

13-Place your arms comfortably by your side, palms facing up. Inhale, pressing your shoulder blades down into the floor lifting up your chest. Roll your shoulder blades back creating a tunnel lengthwise down your back. This will also lift your low back as well. Hold for a count of twenty. Exhale and relax into the floor.

14-Close your eyes and breath normally. Rest in this position for 5 minutes. You are now done with the Primary Flow Pathway.

SECONDARY PATHWAY

The secondary pathway is a more traditional program of specific stretches, isometrics and strengthening exercises. I have set them out starting with stretching and then advancing to isometrics and then strengthening exercise. They are meant to be performed as a complete program that should be done in total because they involve not only shoulder exercises but also ones that strengthen and give flexibility to your core to set you posture correctly. However, feel free to do the exercises that you feel gives you the most benefit.

Begin Secondary Pathway:

Stretching: Hold each position for fifteen seconds, repeat three times.

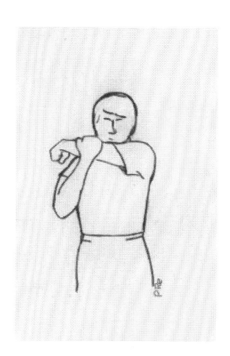

1-Posterior Capsule stretch

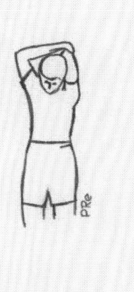

2-Inferior Capsule Stretch

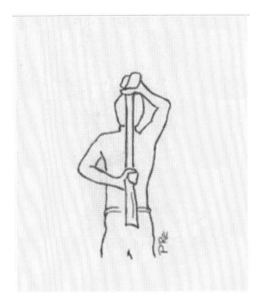

3- Towel-Anterior Capsule Stretch

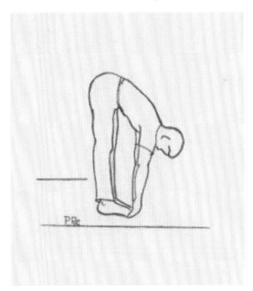

4- Hamstring Stretch

194

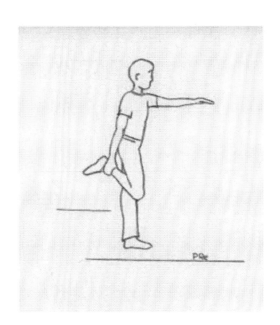

5- Quadriceps Stretch

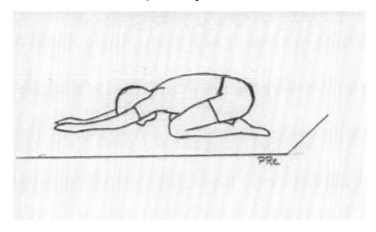

6- Childs Pose

Isometrics: Do each exercise ten times, repeat three times.

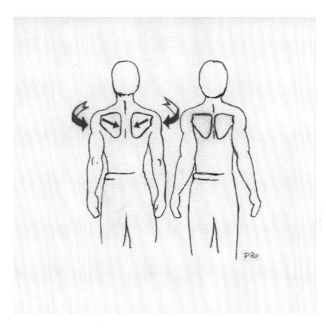

1- Scapular Pinches (crack eggs)

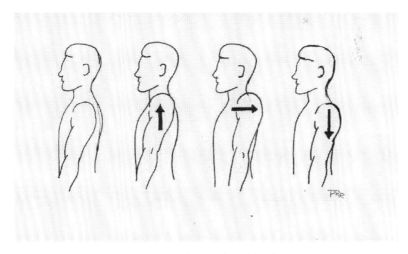

2- Scapular Clock

196

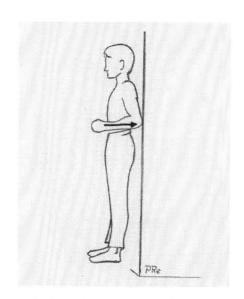

3- Standing Reverse Wall Push ups

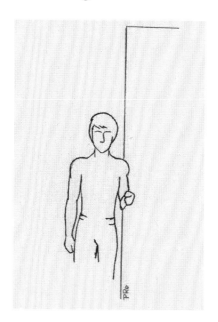

4- Isometric External Rotation

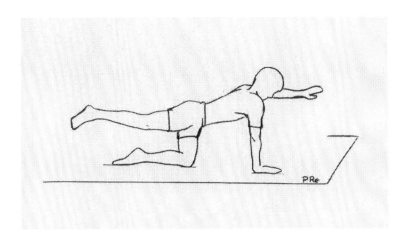

5- All Four Contralateral Upper Arm-Lower Extremity
Extension. Switch sides.

Dynamic Resistive Bands: Do each exercise ten
times, repeat three times.

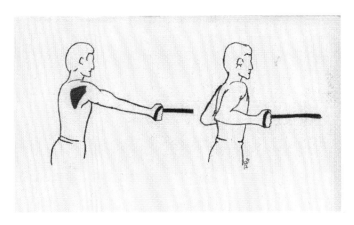

1- Standing Row

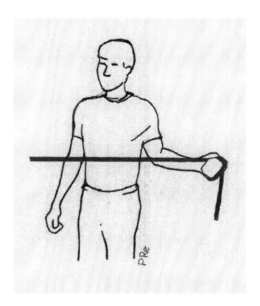

2- Resisted External Rotation

Light Free Weights: Do each exercise ten times, repeat three times. Use 1 or 2 pound weights only. If you don't have weights you can use a can of soup.

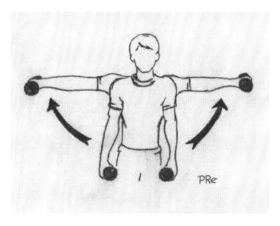

1- Standing Arm Abduction

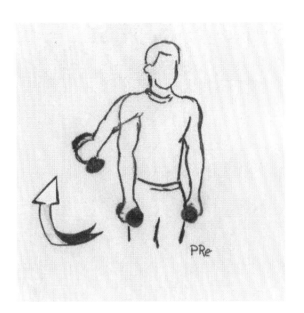

2- Standing 30 Degree Forward Flexion-Thumbs Down

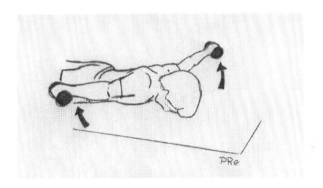

3- Prone Scapular Retraction.

BASIC FIVE

As stated before, I would rather you do five exercises regularly, than to be overwhelmed with some long far reaching program and decide to do nothing. Or if you don't have a lot of time, these simple five exercises focus on scapular retraction and maintaining good scapular position.

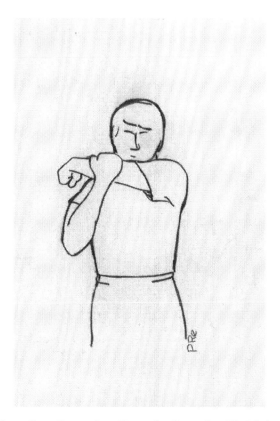

1- Standing Posterior Capsule Stretch: Hold the position for ten seconds. Bring arm by side and perform posterior capsular stretch to the other side, hold for ten seconds. Repeat three times

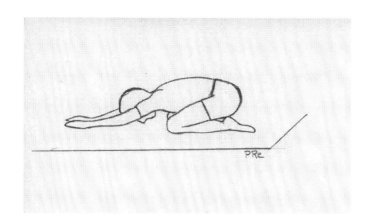

2- Childs Pose: Hold this position for twenty seconds,
repeat three times.

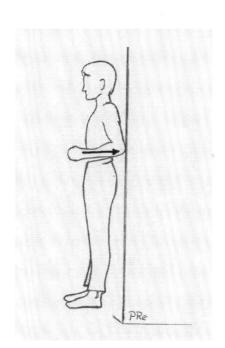

3- Standing Reverse Wall Push Up/Out: Push up/out, hold
for two seconds and release. Do three sets of ten.

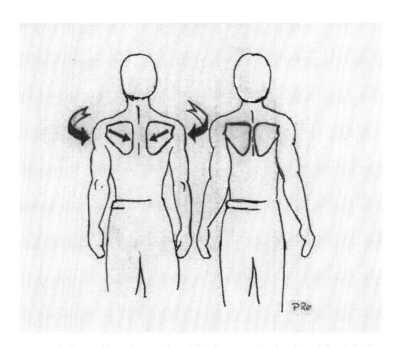

4- Standing Scapular Pinches: Pinch shoulder blades together, hold for two seconds and then release. Do three sets of ten.

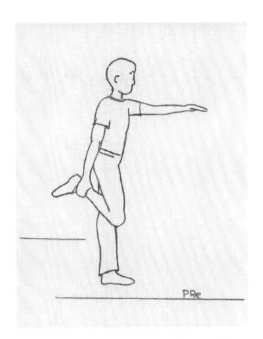

5- Standing Hamstring and Quadriceps Stretch, Core and
Balance: Bend your left knee, bring your left heel to your
buttocks and grab the dorsum of your foot with your left hand.
Extend your right arm forward and reach outward as you lift with
your left hand pulling your left foot/heel and leg higher. Hold for
ten seconds and then release. Do same for right side. Repeat five
times.

FINAL THOUGHTS

I find the shoulder to be one of the most multipurpose, complex and interesting of all our joints. Its unique shape, motion, instability, dynamic stabilization and mechanics make it one of the body's most versatile joints. It has been my good fortune to help patients for more than 18 years, understand their injury and path towards health. It is through education and knowledge of the shoulder that physicians can help patients. Education of the patient is paramount towards recovery and prevention of injury. It is my goal, not only to fix the injury, but educate the patient. Through understanding, the patient can fully participate in recovery. Through understanding, we can help prevent injury.

Please use this book for informational purposes, and as a tool for further inquiry and discussion with your health care provider to address your specific injury.

ABOUT THE AUTHOR

Dr. Paul Re completed his BA in a combined major of Economics and Pre-Medical Studies at Columbia College, Columbia University, and obtained his Medical Degree from Columbia College of Physicians and Surgeons, Columbia University.

He completed his Surgical Internship at Harvard's Fifth Surgical Service, New England Deaconess Hospital and his Orthopedic Surgical Residency at Harvard's Combined Orthopedic Residency, Harvard University. In 1997 he was chosen to be Chief Resident of Orthopedic Surgery at the Massachusetts General Hospital. There he served as clinical Instructor and Associate Trauma Surgeon.

Dr. Re completed three fellowships. His first fellowship was as the Frank E. Stinchfield Fellow in Molecular Biology at New York Orthopedic Hospital, Columbia University. His second fellowship, was the Spine Surgical Fellowship at the Brigham and Woman's Hospital, Harvard University. Dr. Re's final fellowship was in Sports Medicine at New England Medical Center, Tufts University.

Dr. Re is board certified in Orthopedic Surgery, ABOS, and is one of only a few Orthopedic Surgeons who has obtained a second Specialized Board Certification in Sports Medicine, ABOS. He is a member of numerous orthopedic societies and association. Dr. Re has over 20 published articles, chapters and abstracts in peer review journals, text books and national meetings. He has 23 Patent Applications, and has been granted 16 full patents from the United States Patent and Trademark Office USPTO.

Dr. Re has had staff privileges at the Massachusetts General Hospital, Brigham and Women's Hospital, New England Medical Center, and New England Baptist Hospital. At Emerson Hospital he has been appointed Director of Sports Medicine, has served as Associate Chief of Surgery and has been the Chief of Orthopedic Surgery since 2012.

While Dr. Re has expertise in all aspects of orthopedics and orthopedic surgery, his primary love has always been in the complex injuries and treatment of the shoulder.

ABOUT THE EDITOR

Dr. Louis Peter Re is the brother of, and collaborator with Dr. Paul Re.

He is a Board Certified Orthopaedic Surgeon, specializing in treatment of shoulder injuries including Arthroscopic Shoulder Reconstruction. He trained at Columbia University and completed Residency at Yale University School of Medicine where he also served as Clinical Instructor. After his Fellowship at Southern California Orthopaedic Institute, he practiced in Los Angeles before finally settling in New York City working at Riverside Orthopaedics and Sports Medicine Associates, Lenox Hill Hospital and Roosevelt Hospital. More recently he was Assistant Clinical professor at Columbia University College of Physicians and Surgeons. He is currently a Clinical Instructor at Mt. Sinai West in Manhattan.

Made in the USA
Middletown, DE
13 June 2019